ER
Facts

made

Incredibly
Quick!™

M000158189

Staff

Executive Publisher

Judith A. Schilling McCann, RN, MSN

Editorial Director

David Moreau

Clinical Director

Joan M. Robinson, RN, MSN

Senior Art Director

Arlene Putterman

Art Director

Mary Ludwicki

Senior Managing Editor

Jaime Stockslager Buss

Editor

Doris Weinstock

Designer

Lynn Foulk

Illustrator

Bot Roda

Digital Composition Services

Diane Paluba (manager), Joyce Rossi Biletz

Manufacturing

Patricia K. Dorshaw (director), Beth J. Welsh

Editorial Assistants

Megan L. Aldinger, Tara L. Carter-Bell,
Linda K. Ruhf

Indexer

Jaime Stockslager Buss

Printed in China.

ERIIQ010306—010306
ISBN: 1-58255-591-5

Triage
Assessment, Acuity systems, Disaster, Neuro, Cardio, Respir, Musculoskeletal, GI/GU, Skin, Pain

Lab Values
Chemistry, Tumor, CBC, Hematology, Antibiotics, Urine, Cardiac, Crisis, ABGs, CSF

ABCs
CPR, ACLS, Ventilators, Hemodynamics, Pacemakers, ECGs

Meds/IV
Calculations/Conversions, BSA, Transfusions, Antidotes, Therapeutic monitoring, Infusion rates

ER Care
Burns, Pain, Fractures, Head trauma, Heart failure, Seizures, Spinal cord injury, Shock, MI, Stroke, Whiplash, Suicide

Special
Peds, Mat-Neo, Geriatrics

Resource
Vital signs, Conversions, Immunization schedules, Bioterrorism, Brain death, Phone triage, EMTALA, Cultural con

Notes

Primary assessment

Triage is a method of classifying all incoming ED patients, based on their chief complaint and the results of a physical assessment, in order to set priorities of care. It includes primary and secondary assessment.

Parameter	Assessment	Interventions
Airway	• Airway patency	• To open airway, make sure that neck is midline and stabilized; then perform jaw-thrust maneuver.
Breathing	• Respirations (rate, depth, effort) • Breath sounds • Chest wall movement and chest injury • Position of trachea (midline or deviation)	• Administer 100% oxygen with bag-valve mask. • Use airway adjuncts (oral or nasal airway, ET tube, esophageal-tracheal combitube, cricothyrotomy). • Suction as needed. • Remove foreign bodies that may obstruct breathing. • Treat life-threatening conditions.
Circulation	• Pulse and BP • Bleeding or hemorrhage • Capillary refill, color of skin and mucous membranes • Cardiac rhythm	• Administer CPR, medications, and defibrillation or synchronized cardioversion. • Control hemorrhaging with direct pressure or pneumatic devices. • Establish I.V. access and fluid therapy (isotonic fluids and blood). • Treat life-threatening conditions.
Disability	• Neurologic assessment, including LOC, pupils' reactivity to light, and motor and sensory function	• Immobilize cervical spine until X-rays confirm absence of cervical spine injury.
Exposure and environment	• Injuries and environmental exposure (extreme cold or heat)	• Institute warming therapy for hypothermia or cooling therapy for hyperthermia.

Secondary assessment

The mnemonic devices shown below can remind you what questions to ask the patient as part of the secondary assessment.

Subjective data

PQRSTT mnemonic

Provocative/**P**alliative: What provokes the symptom? What makes it better?

Quality/**Q**uantity: What does it feel like? (Use patient's own words.)

Region/**R**adiation: Where is it? Where does it radiate?

Severity: Rate its severity on a scale of 1 to 10.

Timing: How long have you had it? Has it happened before?

Treatment: What treatment worked before arrival in ED?

OLD CART mnemonic

Onset of symptom
Location of symptom
Duration of symptom
Characteristics of symptom (as described by patient)
Aggravating factors
Relieving factors
Treatment before arrival in ED

Objective data

SAMPLE mnemonic

Signs and symptoms
Allergies (if any, as well as reactions)
Medications (including OTC, herbs, vitamins) and last dose
Past medical and surgical history
Last meal
Events leading to injury

Other information to include

• Immunization history (if child) or last tetanus toxoid shot (if adult)
• Primary care physician
• Height and weight
• Date of last menstrual period (if female)
• Method of arrival in ED

Triage acuity systems

Each ED should have its own acuity system.

3-level acuity system

Level	Acuity	Treatment and reassessment time	Sample conditions
1	Emergent	Immediate	Respiratory distress or arrest, coma, poisoning
2	Urgent	20 min-2 hr	Noncardiac chest pain, severe abdominal pain
3	Nonurgent	2-4 hr	Strains and sprains, ear-aches

4-level acuity system

Level	Acuity	Treatment and reassessment time	Sample conditions
1	Emergent	Immediate	Cardiac arrest, anaphylaxis
2	Urgent	15-30 min	Major fractures, sexual assault
3	Semi-urgent	30-60 min	Alcohol intoxication, abdominal pain
4	Nonurgent	1-2 hr	Minor burns or bites

5-level acuity system

Level	Acuity	Treatment and reassessment time	Sample conditions
1	Critical	Immediate	Cardiac arrest, anaphylaxis
2	Unstable	5-15 min	Major fractures, overdose
3	Potentially unstable	30-60 min	Alcohol intoxication, abdominal pain
4	Stable	1-2 hr	Cystitis, minor bites
5	Routine	4 hr	Suture removal

Disaster triage

When a disaster occurs and mass casualties are transported to an emergency department, a system is needed to identify patients who require only minimal care and those likely to die even with maximal efforts.

Minimally injured patients (usually the largest number of victims)

- Place in a separate location outside the emergency department.
- Treat and discharge patients from this area.

Seriously injured but potentially salvageable patients

- Place these patients in an area near the surgical team.
- Assure that a trauma surgeon remains in this area.

Critically injured patients with minimal chance of survival

- Place these patients in a supportive care area.
- Provide sedation and analgesia.
- Refrain from resuscitation efforts.

Special triage populations

Pediatric patients

Because pediatric patients are at high risk for illness and rapid deterioration, always give them special consideration. Be aware of:
• appropriate vital sign ranges
• growth and development issues, including expected height and weight
• duration of the complaint
• hydration status
• immunization status
• allergies
• current medications
• identity of the primary caregiver.

Geriatric patients

Patients older than age 75 are also at increased risk for rapid deterioration. They may also have concurrent medical conditions that can alter assessment findings. Don't assume that abnormal assessment findings are due to aging. Remember that elderly patients may experience:
• decreased cardiac reserve
• depressed sense of pain
• diminished protective airway mechanisms
• decreased resistance to infection
• decreased temperature regulation
• diminished short-term memory.

Non-English speaking patients

When communicating with a non-English speaking patient through a translator, be sure to:
• speak in a normal tone
• speak directly to the patient, not the interpreter
• avoid using complicated medical terminology.

Additionally, observe the patient's nonverbal communication style for eye contact, expressiveness, and ability to understand common signs. Determine the patient's spatial comfort level, particularly in light of his conversation proximity to others and body movement.

Triage documentation

Documentation of the triage assessment and severity rating needs to be clear, concise, and complete. Most hospitals have developed documentation forms or utilize a computerized system. Important documentation elements to include are:

- patient name
- date and time of arrival
- mode of arrival
- triage interview time
- patient age
- prehospital interventions
- first-aid measures
- allergies
- immunization status (pediatric patients)
- cultural assessment, including language spoken
- current medications
- vital signs
- level of pain
- chief complaint
- assessment findings
- medical history
- last menstrual period (for females of childbearing age)
- last tetanus immunization
- fall risk
- triage severity rating
- diagnostic tests initiated
- medications administered
- nursing interventions
- triage reassessment.

NEUROLOGIC SYSTEM
LOC assessment

Classification	Description
Alert	• Follows commands and responds completely and appropriately to stimuli • Oriented to time, place, and person
Lethargy	• Limited spontaneous movement or speech • Easy to arouse by normal speech or touch • Possible disorientation to time, place, or person
Obtundation	• Mild to moderate reduction in arousal • Limited responsiveness to environment • Able to fall asleep easily • Answers questions with minimum response
Stupor	• State of deep sleep or unresponsiveness • Arousable (motor or verbal response) only to vigorous and repeated stimulation • Withdrawal or grabbing response to stimulation
Coma	• No motor or verbal response to any stimuli • No response to noxious stimuli such as deep pain • Unarousable

Pupil measurement

 1 mm

 2 mm

 3 mm

 4 mm

 5mm

 6 mm

 7 mm

 8 mm

 9 mm

Grading deep tendon reflexes

0 absent

+ present but diminished

++ normal

+++ increased but not necessarily abnormal

++++ hyperactive or clonic (involuntary contraction and relaxation of skeletal muscle)

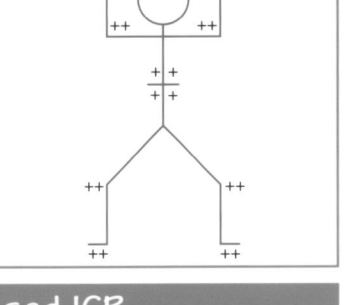

Signs of increased ICP

	Early signs	Late signs
Level of consciousness	• Requires increased stimulation • Subtle orientation loss • Restlessness and anxiety • Sudden quietness	• Unarousable
Pupils	• Pupil changes • One pupil constricts but then dilates (unilateral hippus) • Both pupils sluggish • Unequal pupils	• Pupils fixed and dilated or "blown"
Motor response	• Sudden weakness • Motor changes • Positive pronator drift (with palms up, one hand pronates)	• Profound weakness
Vital signs	• Increased BP	• Increased systolic pressure, profound bradycardia, abnormal respirations

Glasgow Coma Scale

In this test of baseline mental status, a score of 15 indicates that the patient is alert, can follow simple commands, and is oriented to person, place, and time. A decreased score in one or more categories may signal an impending neurologic crisis. A score of 7 or less indicates severe neurologic damage.

Test	Score	Patient response
Eye-opening response		
Spontaneously	4	Opens eyes spontaneously
To speech	3	Opens eyes when instructed
To pain	2	Opens eyes only to painful stimulus
None	1	Doesn't open eyes to stimuli
Motor response		
Obeys	6	Shows two fingers when asked
Localizes	5	Reaches toward painful stimulus and tries to remove it
Withdraws	4	Moves away from painful stimulus
Abnormal flexion	3	Assumes a decorticate posture
Abnormal extension	2	Assumes a decerebrate posture
None	1	No response; just lies flaccid
Verbal response (to question "What year is this?")		
Oriented	5	States correct date
Confused	4	States incorrect year
Inappropriate words	3	Replies randomly with incorrect words
Incomprehensible	2	Moans or screams
No response	1	No response
Total score		

Dermatomes

Knowledge of dermatomes is useful to localize neurologic lesions. The two illustrations here demonstrate the patterns of dermatomes on the body.

Anterior

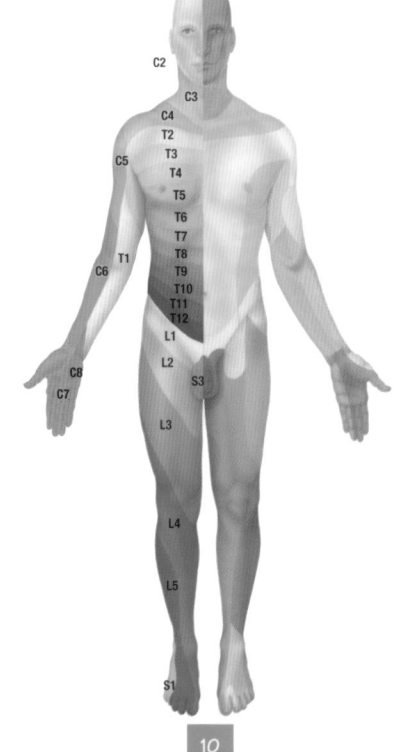

Posterior

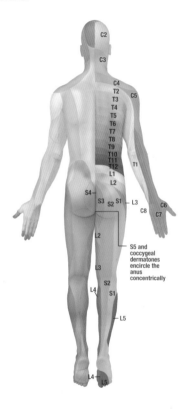

C2
C3
C4
T2
T3
C5
T4
T5
T6
T7
T8
T9
T10
T11
T12
T1
L1
L2
S4
S3 S2 S1 L3
C8
C7
C6
L2
S5 and
coccygeal
dermatones
encircle the
anus
concentrically
L3
S2
L4 S1
L5
L4 L5

Heart sound sites

When auscultating for heart sounds, place the stethoscope over the four sites circled below.

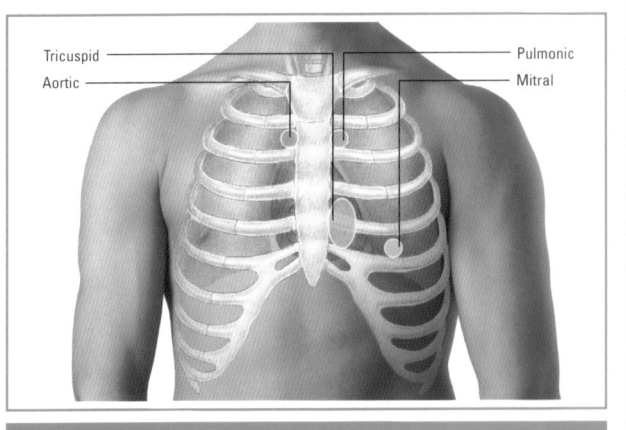

Tricuspid — — Pulmonic
Aortic — — Mitral

Grading murmurs

Use the system outlined below to describe the intensity of a murmur:
• Grade I is a barely audible murmur.
• Grade II is audible but quiet and soft.
• Grade III is moderately loud, without a thrust or thrill.
• Grade IV is loud, with a thrill.
• Grade V is very loud, with a thrust or a thrill.
• Grade VI is loud enough to be heard before the stethoscope comes into contact with the chest.

When recording your findings, use Roman numerals as part of a fraction, always with VI as the denominator. For instance, a grade III murmur would be recorded as "grade III/VI."

Capillary refill

Normal: < 3 sec
Abnormal: > 3 sec

Grading pulses

Pulses should be regular in rhythm and strength. Check carotid, brachial, radial, femoral, popliteal, posterior tibial, and dorsal pedis pulses. Grade them using the numerical scale below.

4+ =	bounding
3+ =	increased
2+ =	normal
1+ =	weak
0 =	absent

Jugular vein distention

Normal: jugular vein < 1½" (4 cm) in diameter
Jugular vein distention: > 1½" in diameter

Edema scale

0	None observed
+1	Minimal (< 2 mm)
+2	Depression 2–4 mm
+3	Depression 5–8 mm
+4	Depression > 8 mm

Assessment landmarks

Anterior view

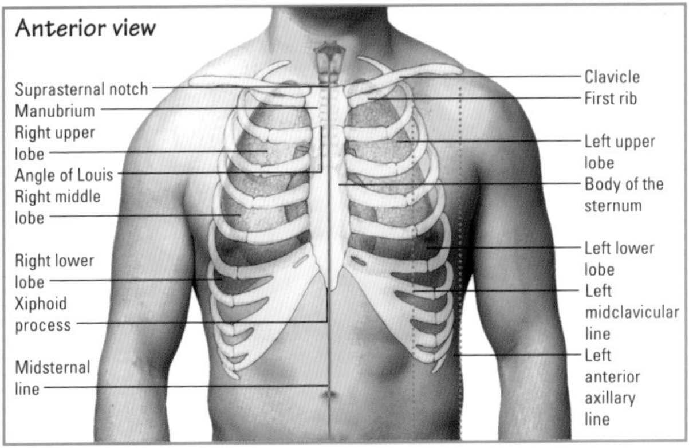

- Suprasternal notch
- Manubrium
- Right upper lobe
- Angle of Louis
- Right middle lobe
- Right lower lobe
- Xiphoid process
- Midsternal line
- Clavicle
- First rib
- Left upper lobe
- Body of the sternum
- Left lower lobe
- Left midclavicular line
- Left anterior axillary line

Posterior view

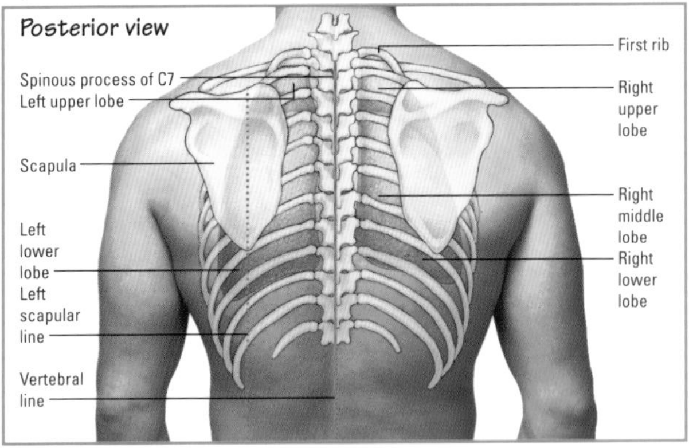

- Spinous process of C7
- Left upper lobe
- Scapula
- Left lower lobe
- Left scapular line
- Vertebral line
- First rib
- Right upper lobe
- Right middle lobe
- Right lower lobe

Respiratory assessment

Inspection	Chest configuration, tracheal position, chest symmetry, skin condition, nostril flaring, accessory muscle use, respiratory rate and pattern, cyanosis, clubbing of fingers
Palpation	Crepitus, pain, tactile fremitus, scars, lumps, lesions, ulcerations, chest wall symmetry and expansion
Percussion	Resonance (normal), hyperresonance, dullness, tympany
Auscultation	Four types of breath sounds over normal lungs: tracheal, bronchial, bronchovesicular, and vesicular

Abnormal breath sounds

Sound	Description
Crackles	Light crackling, popping, intermittent nonmusical sounds — like hairs being rubbed together — heard on inspiration or expiration
Pleural friction rub	Low-pitched, continual, superficial, squeaking or grating sound — like pieces of sandpaper being rubbed together — heard on inspiration and expiration
Rhonchi	Low-pitched, monophonic snoring sounds heard primarily on expiration but also throughout the respiratory cycle
Stridor	High-pitched, monophonic crowing sound heard on inspiration; louder in the neck than in the chest wall
Wheezes	High-pitched, continual musical or whistling sound heard primarily on expiration but sometimes also on inspiration

MUSCULOSKELETAL SYSTEM

Normal findings

Inspection

- No gross deformities
- Symmetrical body parts
- Good body alignment
- No involuntary movements
- Smooth gait
- Active range of motion and no pain in all muscles and joints
- No swelling or inflammation visible in muscles or joints
- Equal bilateral limb length and symmetrical muscle mass

Palpation

- Normal shape, with no swelling or tenderness
- Equal bilateral muscle tone, texture, and strength
- No involuntary contractions or twitching
- Equally strong bilateral pulses

Grading muscle strength

5/5: Normal: patient moves joint through full range of motion (ROM) and against gravity with full resistance

4/5: Good: patient completes ROM against gravity with moderate resistance

3/5: Fair: patient completes ROM against gravity only

2/5: Poor: patient completes full ROM with gravity eliminated (passive motion)

1/5: Trace: patient's attempt at muscle contraction is palpable but without joint movement

0/5: Zero: no evidence of muscle contraction

The 5 P's of musculoskeletal injury

To assess a musculoskeletal injury, remember the 5 P's.

Pain

Ask the patient if he feels pain.

Paresthesia

Assess for loss of sensation.

Paralysis

Assess whether the patient can move the affected area.

Pallor

Paleness, discoloration, and coolness on the injured side may indicate neurovascular compromise.

Pulse

Check all pulses distal to the injury site.

Abdominal quadrants

Right upper quadrant

- Right lobe of the liver
- Gallbladder
- Pylorus
- Duodenum
- Head of the pancreas
- Hepatic flexure of the colon
- Portions of the transverse and ascending colon

Left upper quadrant

- Left lobe of the liver
- Stomach
- Body of the pancreas
- Splenic flexure of the colon
- Portions of the transverse and descending colon

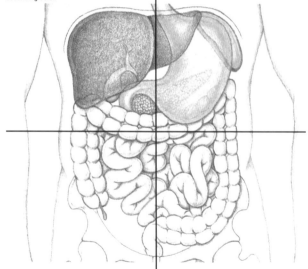

Right lower quadrant

- Cecum and appendix
- Portion of the ascending colon

Left lower quadrant

- Sigmoid colon
- Portion of the descending colon

GI and GU assessment

Inspection

- *GI:* Abdominal symmetry, shape, and contour; bumps; bulges; bruises; masses; striae; dilated veins; scars; movement and pulsations; distention; skin tightness; glistening
- *GU:* Inflammation or discharge from urethral meatus

Palpation

- *GI:* Abdominal size, shape, and position; tenderness of major organs; masses; fluid accumulation
- *GU:* Kidneys and bladder

Auscultation

- *GI:* Bowel motility; underlying vessels and organs; bowel sounds (normal, hypoactive, or hyperactive); bruits, venous hum, or friction rub
- *GU:* Renal arteries (with bell in left and right upper abdominal quadrants)

Percussion

- *GI:* Tympany, dullness, size and location of abdominal organs, excessive accumulation of fluid and air
Note: Don't percuss the abdomen if an abdominal aortic aneurysm or a transplanted abdominal organ is present.
- *GU:* Kidneys for tenderness; bladder for position and contents

INTEGUMENTARY SYSTEM

Assessing skin characteristics

Color: Note bruising, discoloration, erythema, pallor, duskiness, jaundice, or cyanosis.
Texture: Note mobility, thickness, thinness, roughness, smoothness, or fragility.
Turgor: After squeezing skin on forearm, note if it returns to regular shape quickly, returns slowly, or leaves a tented shape.
Moisture: Note excessive dryness, moisture, or diaphoresis.
Temperature: Note generalized or localized coolness or warmth.
Lesions: Note vascular changes, hemangiomas, telangiectases, petechiae, purpura, ecchymosis, and any skin lesions.

PAIN ASSESSMENT

PQRSTT mnemonic

The PQRSTT mnemonic below is a useful tool in assessing pain:
Provokes/**P**oint: What provokes or exacerbates the pain? What makes it better? Point to where you feel the pain.
Quality: What does it feel like? Sharp? Dull? Stabbing? Burning? Crushing?
Radiation/**R**elief: Where is the pain? Where does it radiate? What relieves the pain?
Severity: Rate the pain's severity on a scale of 1 to 10 (or use another pain-rating scale, depending on the patient).
Time: When did the pain start? How long did it last?
Treatment: What treatment alleviates it?

Other questions to ask

• Is deep inspiration painful?
• Were you performing an activity at the onset of pain?
• Any prior history of pain? If so, is current pain the same as before or different?
• Any recent trauma?
• Any other symptoms associated with the pain, such as nausea and vomiting?
• Any effects on lifestyle, such as appetite, sleep, relationships, emotions, and work?
• Any medications or allergies?

Numeric pain rating scale

A numeric rating scale can help the patient quantify his pain. Have him choose a number from 0 (indicating no pain) to 10 (indicating the worst pain imaginable) to reflect his current pain level. He can either circle the number on the scale itself or verbally state the number that best describes his pain.

| No pain | 0 | 1 | 2 | 3 | 4 | 5 | 6 | 7 | 8 | 9 | 10 | Pain as bad as it can be |

Visual analog scale

To use the visual analog scale, ask the patient to place a mark on the scale to indicate his current level of pain.

No pain |—————————————————————————| Pain as bad as it can be

Wong-Baker FACES Pain Rating Scale

A pediatric patient or an adult patient with language difficulties may not be able to express the pain he's feeling. In such cases, use the pain intensity scale below. Ask the patient to choose the face that best represents the severity of his pain on a scale from 0 to 10.

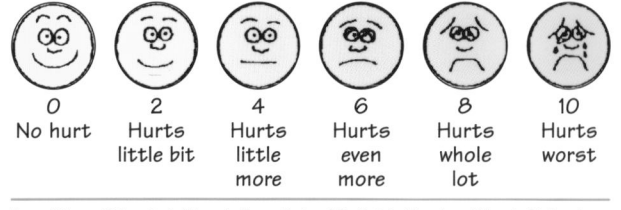

| 0 | 2 | 4 | 6 | 8 | 10 |
| No hurt | Hurts little bit | Hurts little more | Hurts even more | Hurts whole lot | Hurts worst |

From Wong, D.L., et al. *Wong's Essentials of Pediatric Nursing*, 6th ed. St. Louis: Mosby–Year Book, Inc., 2001. Reprinted with permission.

Common pain medications for adults

Opioids

Drug	Oral dosage	Parenteral dosage
codeine	15-60 mg q 4-6 hr	phosphate: 15-60 mg subQ, I.M., or I.V. q 4-6 hr
hydromorphone	2-4 mg q 4-6 hr	1-4 mg subQ, I.M., or I.V. (over 2-5 min) q 4-6 hr
meperidine	50-150 mg q 3-4 hr	50-150 mg subQ or I.M. q 3-4 hr
methadone	2.5-10 mg q 3-4 hr	2.5-4 mg subQ or I.M. q 3-4 hr
morphine	5-30 mg q 4 hr	5-20 mg subQ or I.M. q 4 hr or 2.5-15 mg I.V. q 4 hr
oxycodone	5 mg q 6 hr	N/A
oxymorphone	N/A	0.5 mg I.V., or 1 to 1.5 mg subQ or I.M. q 4-6 hr
propoxyphene	HCl: 65 mg q 4 hr napsylate: 100 mg q 4 hr	N/A
tramadol	50-100 mg P.O. q 4-6 hr	N/A

NSAIDs

Drug	Typical dosage
celecoxib	400 mg P.O. daily
diclofenac	50 mg P.O. q 8 hr
diflunisal	Loading dose of 500-1,000 mg P.O., then 500 mg P.O. q 12 hr
etodolac	200-400 mg P.O. q 6-8 hr
fenoprofen	200 mg P.O. q 4-6 hr
ibuprofen	400 mg P.O. q 4-6 hr
indomethacin	25 mg P.O. q 8-12 hr
ketoprofen	25-50 mg P.O. q 6-8 hr
ketorolac	30 mg I.M. or I.V. q 6 hr
nabumetone	1 g P.O. daily
naproxen	250-500 mg P.O. q 12 hr
piroxicam	20 mg P.O. daily
sulindac	150 mg P.O. q 12 hr
valdecoxib	10 mg P.O. daily

Nonopioid analgesics

Drug	Oral dosage
acetaminophen	325-650 mg q 4-6 hr
aspirin	325-650 mg P.O. q 4 hr

Combination opioid analgesics

Drug	Brand names	Dosage
acetaminophen and propoxyphene napsylate	Darvocet	1 tablet q 4 hr
acetaminophen and hydrocodone	Lortab, Vicodin	1-2 tablets q 4 hr
acetaminophen and oxycodone	Percocet, Tylox	1-2 tablets q 4-6 hr
aspirin, oxycodone HCl, and oxycodone terephthalate	Percodan	1 tablet q 6 hr
acetaminophen and codeine phosphate	Tylenol with codeine #2	1-2 tablets q 4 hr
	Tylenol with codeine #3	1-2 tablets q 4 hr
	Tylenol with codeine #4	1 tablet q 4 hr

Comprehensive metabolic panel

Test	Conventional units	SI units
Albumin	3.5-5 g/dl	35-50 g/L
Alkaline phosphatase	45-115 units/L	45-115 units/L
ALT	Male: 10-40 units/L	0.17-0.68 µkat/L
	Female: 7-35 units/L	0.12-0.60 µkat/L
AST	12-31 units/L	0.21-0.53 µkat/L
Bilirubin, total	0.2-1 mg/dl	3.5-17 µmol/L
BUN	8-20 mg/dl	2.9-7.5 mmol/L
Calcium	8.2-10.2 mg/dl	2.05-2.54 mmol/L
Carbon dioxide	22-26 mEq/L	22-26 mmol/L
Chloride	100-108 mEq/L	100-108 mmol/L
Creatinine	Male: 0.8-1.2 mg/dl	62-115 µmol/L
	Female: 0.6-0.9 mg/dl	53-97 µmol/L
Glucose	70-100 mg/dl	3.9-6.1 mmol/L
Potassium	3.5-5 mEq/L	3.5-5 mmol/L
Protein, total	6.3-8.3 g/dl	64-83 g/L
Sodium	135-145 mEq/L	135-145 mmol/L

Lipid panel

Test	Conventional units	SI units
Total cholesterol	< 200 mg/dl	< 5.18 mmol/L
HDL cholesterol	≥ 60 mg/dl	≥ 1.55 mmol/L
LDL cholesterol	< 130 mg/dl	< 3.36 mmol/L
VLDL cholesterol	< 130 mg/dl	< 3.4 mmol/L
Triglycerides	< 150 mg/dl	< 1.7 mmol/L

Thyroid panel

Test	Conventional units	SI units
T_3	80-200 ng/dl	1.2-3 nmol/L
T_4, free	0.9-2.3 ng/dl	10-30 nmol/L
T_4, total	5-13.5 mcg/dl	60-165 mmol/L
TSH	0.4-4.2 mIU/L	0.4-4.2 mIU/L

Other chemistry tests

Test	Conventional units	SI units
A/G ratio	3.4-4.8 g/dl	34-38 g/dl
Ammonia	< 50 ng/dl	< 36 µmol/L
Amylase	26-102 units/L	0.4-1.74 µkat/L
Anion gap	8-14 mEq/L	8-14 mmol/L
Bilirubin, direct	< 0.5 mg/dl	< 6.8 µmol/L
Calcitonin	Male: < 16 pg/ml	< 16 ng/L
	Female: < 8 pg/ml	< 8 ng/L
Calcium, ionized	4.65-5.28 mg/dl	1.1-1.25 mmol/L
Cortisol	a.m.: 7-25 mcg/dl	0.2-0.7 µmol/L
	p.m.: 2-14 mcg/dl	0.06-0.39 µmol/L
C-reactive protein	< 0.8 mg/dl	< 8 mg/L
Ferritin	Male: 20-300 ng/ml	20-300 mcg/L
	Female: 20-120 ng/ml	20-120 mcg/L
Folate	1.8-20 ng/ml	4.5-45.3 nmol/L
GGT	Male: 7-47 units/L	0.12-1.80 µkat/L
	Female: 5-25 units/L	0.08-0.42 µkat/L
Hb_{A1c}	4%-7%	0.04-0.07
Homocysteine	< 12 µmol/L	< 12 µmol/L
Iron	Male: 65-175 mcg/dl	11.6-31.3 µmol/L
	Female: 50-170 mcg/dl	9-30.4 µmol/L
Iron-binding capacity	250-400 mcg/dl	45-72 µmol/L
Lactic acid	0.5-2.2 mEq/L	0.5-2.2 mmol/L
Lipase	10-73 units/L	0.17-1.24 µkat/L
Magnesium	1.3-2.2 mg/dl	0.65-1.05 mmol/L
Osmolality	275-295 mOsm/kg	275-295 mOsm/kg

Test	Conventional units	SI units
Phosphate	2.7-4.5 mg/dl	0.87-1.45 mmol/L
Prealbumin	19-38 mg/dl	190-380 mg/L
Uric acid	Male: 3.4-7 mg/dl	202-416 µmol/L
	Female: 2.3-6 mg/dl	143-357 µmol/L

Tumor markers

Test	Conventional units	SI units
Alpa-fetoprotein	< 40 ng/ml	< 40 mcg/L
CA 15-3	< 30 units/ml	< 30 kU/L
CA 19-9	< 37 units/ml	< 37 kU/L
CA 27-29	≤ 38 units/ml	≤ 38 kU/L
CA 125	< 35 units/ml	< 35 kU/L
Carcinoembryonic antigen	< 2.5-5 ng/ml	< 2.5-5 mcg/L
Human chorionic gonadotropin	< 2 ng/ml	< 2 mcg/L
Neuron-specific enolase	< 12.5 mcg/ml	—
PSA	Age 40-49: ≤ 2.5 ng/ml	≤ 2.5 mcg/L
	Age 50-59: ≤ 3.5 ng/ml	≤ 3.5 mcg/L
	Age 60-69: ≤ 4.5 ng/ml	≤ 4.5 mcg/L
	Age 70+: ≤ 6.5 ng/ml	≤ 6.5 mcg/L

Complete blood count with differential

Test	Conventional units	SI units
Hemoglobin	Male: 14-17.4 g/dl	140-174 g/L
	Female: 12-16 g/dl	120-160 g/L
Hematocrit	Male: 42%-52%	0.42-0.52
	Female: 36%-48%	0.36-0.48
RBC	Male: 4.2-5.4 × 10^6/mm^3	4.2-5.4 × 10^{12}/L
	Female: 3.6-5 × 10^6/mm^3	3.6-5 × 10^{12}/L
MCH	26-34 pg/cell	0.40-0.53 fmol/cell
MCHC	32-36 g/dl	320-360 g/L

(continued)

Complete blood count with differential *(continued)*

Test	Conventional units	SI units
MCV	82-98 mm^3	82-98 fL
WBC	4,000-10,000/cells/mm^3	4-10 $\times$ 10^9/L
Bands	0%-5%	0.03-0.08
Basophils	0%-1%	0-0.01
Eosinophils	1%-4%	0.01-0.04
Lymphocytes	25%-40%	0.25-0.40
Monocytes	2%-8%	0.02-0.08
Neutrophils	54%-75%	0.54-0.75
Platelets	140,000-400,000/mm^3	140-400 x 10^9/L

Coagulation studies

Test	Conventional units	SI units
ACT	107 sec $\pm$ 13 sec	107 sec $\pm$ 13 sec
Bleeding time	3-6 min	3-6 min
D-dimer	< 250 mcg/L	< 1.37 nmol/L
Fibrinogen	200-400 mg/dl	2-4 g/L
INR (target therapeutic)	2.0-3.0	2.0-3.0
Plasminogen	80%-130%	—
PT	10-14 sec	10-14 sec
PTT	21-35 sec	21-35 sec
Thrombin time	10-15 sec	10-15 sec

Other hematology tests

Test	Conventional units	SI units
Erythrocyte sedimentation rate	Male: 0-10 mm/hr Female: 0-20 mm/hr	0-10 mm/hr 0-20 mm/hr
Pyruvate kinase	2.8-8.8 units/g Hb	46.7-146.7 µkat/g Hb

Antibiotic peaks and troughs

Test	Conventional units	SI units
Amikacin		
Peak	20-30 mcg/ml	34-52 µmol/L
Trough	1-4 mcg/ml	2-7 µmol/L
Chloramphenicol		
Peak	15-25 mcg/ml	46.4-77 µmol/L
Trough	5-15 mcg/ml	15.5-46.4 µmol/L
Gentamycin		
Peak	4-8 mcg/ml	8.4-16.7 µmol/L
Trough	1-2 mcg/ml	2.1-4.2 µmol/L
Tobramycin		
Peak	4-8 mcg/ml	8.6-17.1 µmol/L
Trough	1-2 mcg/ml	2.1-4.3 µmol/L
Vancomycin		
Peak	25-40 mcg/ml	14-27 µmol/L
Trough	5-10 mcg/ml	3.4-6.8 µmol/L

Urine tests

Test	Conventional units	SI units
Urinalysis		
Appearance	Clear to slightly hazy	—
Color	Straw to dark yellow	—
pH	4.5-8	—
Specific gravity	1.005-1.035	—
Glucose	None	—
Protein	None	—
RBCs	None or rare	—
WBCs	None or rare	—
Osmolality	50-1,400 mOsm/kg	—

Cardiac biomarkers

Protein	Conventional units	SI units	Initial evaluation	Peak	Time to return to normal
Troponin-I	< 0.35 mcg/L	< 0.35 mcg/L	4-6 hr	12 hr	3-10 days
Troponin-T	< 0.1 mcg/L	< 0.1 mcg/L	4-8 hr	12-48 hr	7-10 days
Myoglobin	< 55 ng/ml	< 55 mcg/L	2-4 hr	8-10 hr	24 hr
Hs-CRP	0.020-0.800 mg/dl	0.2-8 mg/L	—	—	Depends on degree of inflammation

Enzyme	Conventional units	SI units	Initial evaluation	Peak	Time to return to normal
CK	Male: 55-170 units/L Female: 30-135 units/L	0.94-2.89 μkat/L 0.51-2.3 μkat/L	—	—	—
CK-MB	< 5%	< 0.05	4-8 hr	12-24 hr	72-96 hr
LD	140-280 units/L	2.34-4.68 μkat/L	2-5 days	—	10 days

Hormone	Conventional units	SI units	Initial evaluation	Peak	Time to return to normal
BNP	< 100 pg/ml	< 100 ng/L	—	—	Depends on severity of heart failure

Crisis laboratory values

Test	Low value	High value
Calcium, serum	< 6 mg/dl (SI: < 1.5 mmol/L)	> 13 mg/dl (SI: > 3.2 mmol/L)
Carbon dioxide	< 10 mEq/L (SI: < 10 mmol/L)	> 40 mEq/L (SI: > 40 mmol/L)
Creatinine, serum	—	> 4 mg/dl (SI: > 353.6 μmol/L)
Glucose, blood	< 40 mg/dl (SI: 2.2 mmol/L)	> 300 mg/dl (SI: > 16.6 mmol/L)
Hb	< 8 g/dl (SI: < 80 g/L)	> 18 g/dl (SI: > 180 g/L)
INR	—	> 3.0
$Paco_2$	< 20 mm Hg (SI: < 2.7 kPa)	> 70 mm Hg (SI: > 9.3 kPa)
Pao_2	< 50 mm Hg (SI: < 6.7 kPa)	—
pH, blood	< 7.2 (SI: < 7.2)	> 7.6 (SI: > 7.6)
Platelet count	< 50,000/mm^3	> 500,000/mm^3
Potassium, serum	< 3 mEq/L (SI: < 3 mmol/L)	> 6 mEq/L (SI: > 6 mmol/L)
PT	—	> 14 sec (SI: > 14 s); for patient on warfarin, > 20 sec (SI: > 20 s)
PTT	—	> 40 sec (SI: > 40 s); for patient on heparin, > 70 sec (SI: > 70 s)
Sodium, serum	< 120 mEq/L (SI: < 120 mmol/L)	> 160 mEq/L (SI: > 160 mmol/L)
WBC count	< 2,000/mm^3 (SI: < 2 × 10^9/L)	> 20,000/mm^3 (SI: > 20 × 10^9/L)

Arterial blood gas values

Disorder	ABG findings	Possible causes
Respiratory acidosis (excess CO_2 retention)	• pH < 7.35 • HCO_3^- > 26 mEq/L (if compensating) • $Paco_2$ > 45 mm Hg	• Central nervous system depression from drugs, injury, or disease • Hypoventilation from respiratory, cardiac, musculoskeletal, or neuromuscular disease
Respiratory alkalosis (excess CO_2 loss)	• pH > 7.45 • HCO_3^- < 22 mEq/L (if compensating) • $Paco_2$ < 35 mm Hg	• Hyperventilation due to anxiety, pain, or improper ventilator settings • Respiratory stimulation from drugs, disease, hypoxia, fever, or high room temperature • Gram-negative bacteremia
Metabolic acidosis (HCO_3^- loss or acid retention)	• pH < 7.35 • HCO_3^- < 22 mEq/L • $Paco_2$ < 35 mm Hg (if compensating)	• Depletion of HCO_3^- from renal disease, diarrhea, or small-bowel fistulas • Excessive production of organic acids from hepatic disease, endocrine disorders such as diabetes mellitus, hypoxia, shock, or drug toxicity • Inadequate excretion of acids due to renal disease
Metabolic alkalosis (HCO_3^- retention or acid loss)	• pH > 7.45 • HCO_3^- > 26 mEq/L • $Paco_2$ > 45 mm Hg (if compensating)	• Loss of hydrochloric acid from prolonged vomiting or gastric suctioning • Loss of potassium from increased renal excretion (as in diuretic therapy) or corticosteroid overdose • Excessive alkali ingestion

CSF analysis

Test	Normal	Abnormal	Implications
Pressure	50-180 mm H_2O	Increased Decrease	Increased ICP Spinal subarachnoid obstruction above puncture site
Appearance	Clear, colorless	Cloudy Xanthochromic or bloody Brown, orange, or yellow	Infection Subarachnoid, intracerebral, or intraventricular hemorrhage; spinal cord obstruction; traumatic lumbar puncture (only in initial specimen) Elevated protein levels, RBC breakdown (blood present for at least 3 days)
Protein	15-50 mg/dl (SI: 0.15-0.5 g/L)	Marked increase Marked decrease	Tumors, trauma, hemorrhage, diabetes mellitus, polyneuritis, blood in CSF Rapid CSF production
Gamma globulin	3%-12% of total protein	Increase	Demyelinating disease, neurosyphilis, Guillain-Barré syndrome
Glucose	50-80 mg/dl (SI: 2.8- 4.4 mmol/L)	Increase Decrease	Systemic hyperglycemia Systemic hypoglycemia, bacterial or fungal infection, meningitis, mumps, postsubarachnoid hemorrhage

(continued)

CSF analysis (continued)

Test	Normal	Abnormal	Implications
Cell count	0-5 WBCs	Increase	Active disease: meningitis, acute infection, onset of chronic illness, tumor, abscess, infarction, demyelinating disease
	No RBCs	RBCs	Hemorrhage or traumatic lumbar puncture
VDRL	Nonreactive	Positive	Neurosyphilis
Chloride	118-130 mEq/L (SI: 118 to 130 mmol/L)	Decrease	Infected meninges
Gram stain	No organisms	Gram-positive or gram-negative organisms	Bacterial meningitis

CPR

Before beginning basic life support, CPR, or rescue breathing, activate the appropriate code team.

Adult or adolescent

Check for unresponsiveness	Gently shake and shout, "Are you okay?"
Call for help/call 911	Immediately call 911 for help. If a second rescuer is available, send him to get help or an AED and initiate CPR if indicated. If asphyxial arrest is likely, perform 5 cycles (about 2 min) of CPR before activating EMS.
Position patient	Place patient in supine position on hard, flat surface.
Open airway	Use head-tilt, chin-lift maneuver unless contraindicated by trauma.
If you suspect trauma	Open airway using jaw-thrust method if trauma is suspected.
Check for adequate breathing	Look, listen, and feel for 10 sec.
Perform ventilations	Do 2 breaths initially that make the chest rise at 1 second/breath; then 1 every 5 to 6 sec.
If chest doesn't rise	Reposition and reattempt ventilation. Several attempts may be necessary.
Check pulse	Palpate the carotid for no more than 10 sec.
Start compressions	
Placement	Place both hands, one atop the other, on lower half of sternum between the nipples, with elbows locked; use straight up-and-down motion without losing contact with chest.
Depth	One-third depth of chest or 1½" to 2"
Rate	100/min
Comp-to-vent ratio	30:2 (if intubated, continuous chest compressions at a rate of 100/min without pauses for ventilation; ventilation at 8 to 10 breaths/min)
Check pulse	Check after 2 min of CPR and as appropriate thereafter. Minimize interruptions in chest compressions.
Use AED	Apply as soon as available and follow prompts. Provide 2 min of CPR after first shock is delivered before activating AED to reanalyze rhythm and attempt another shock.

CPR

Child (1 year to onset of adolescence or puberty)

Check for unresponsiveness	Gently shake and shout, "Are you okay?"
Call for help/call 911	Call after 2 min of CPR. Call immediately for witnessed collapse.
Position patient	Place patient in a supine position on a hard, flat surface.
Open airway	Use head-tilt, chin-lift maneuver unless contraindicated by trauma.
If you suspect trauma	Open airway using jaw-thrust method if trauma is suspected.
Check breathing	Look, listen, and feel for 10 sec.
Perform ventilations	Do two breaths initially that make the chest rise at 1 sec/breath; then one every 3 to 5 sec.
If chest doesn't rise	Reposition and reattempt ventilation. Several attempts may be necessary.
Check pulse	Palpate the carotid or femoral for no more than 10 sec.
Start compressions	
Placement	Place heel of one hand or place both hands, one atop the other, with elbows locked, on lower half of sternum between the nipples.
Depth	1/3 to 1/2 depth of the chest
Rate	100/min
Comp:Vent ratio	30:2 (if intubated, continuous chest compressions at a rate of 100/min without pauses for ventilation; ventilation at 8 to 10 breaths/min)
Check pulse	Check after 2 min of CPR and as appropriate thereafter. Minimize interruptions in chest compressions.
AED	Use as soon as available and follow prompts. Use child pads and child system for child age 1 to 8 years. Provide 2 min of CPR after first shock is delivered before activating AED to reanalyze rhythm and attempt another shock.

CPR

Infant (0 to 1 year)

Check unresponsiveness	Gently shake and flick bottom of foot and call out name.
Call for help/call 911	Call after 2 min of CPR. Call immediately for witnessed collapse.
Position patient	Place patient in a supine position on a hard, flat surface.
Open airway	Use head-tilt, chin-lift maneuver unless contraindicated by trauma. Don't hyperextend the neck.
If you suspect trauma	Open airway using jaw-thrust method if trauma is suspected.
Check breathing	Look, listen, and feel for 10 sec.
Perform ventilations	Do two breaths initially that make the chest rise at 1 sec/breath; then one every 3 to 5 sec.
If chest doesn't rise	Reposition and reattempt ventilation. Several attempts may be necessary.
Check pulse	Palpate brachial or femoral pulse for no more than 10 sec.
Start compressions	
Placement	Place two fingers 1 fingerwidth below nipples.
Depth	⅓ to ½ depth of the chest
Rate	100/min
Comp:Vent ratio	30:2 (if intubated, continuous chest compressions at a rate of 100/min without pauses for ventilation; ventilation at 8 to 10 breaths/min)
Check pulse	Check after 2 min of CPR and as appropriate thereafter. Minimize interruptions in chest compression.

Choking

Adult or child older than age 1

Symptoms

- Grabbing throat with hand
- Inability to speak
- Weak, ineffective coughing
- High-pitched sounds while inhaling

Interventions

1. Ask the person, "Are you choking? Can you speak?" Assess for airway obstruction. Don't intervene if the person is coughing forcefully and can speak; a strong cough can dislodge the object.

2. Stand behind the person and wrap your arms around the waist. (If the person is pregnant or obese, wrap your hands around the chest.)

3. Make a fist with one hand, and place the thumb side of your fist just above the person's navel and well below the sternum.

4. Grasp your fist with your other hand.

5. Perform quick, upward and inward thrusts with your fist (perform chest thrusts for pregnant or obese persons).

6. Continue thrusts until the object is dislodged or the victim loses consciousness.

If the victim loses consciousness, activate the emergency response system and provide CPR. Each time you open the airway to deliver rescue breaths, look in the mouth and remove any object you see. Never perform a blind finger sweep.

Choking

Infant (younger than 1 year)

Symptoms

- Inability to cry or make much sound
- Weak, ineffective coughing
- Soft or high-pitched sounds while inhaling
- Bluish skin color

Interventions

1. Assess that the airway is obstructed. Don't perform the next two steps if the infant is coughing forcefully or has a strong cry.
2. Lay the infant face down along your forearm. Hold his chest in your hand and his jaw with your fingers. Point the infant's head downward, lower than the body. Use your thigh or lap for support.
3. Give five quick, forceful blows between the infant's shoulder blades using the heel of your free hand.

After five blows

1. Turn the infant face up.
2. Place two fingers on the middle of the infant's sternum just below the nipples.
3. Give five quick thrusts down, compressing the chest ½″ to 1″ (⅓ to ½ the depth of the chest).
4. Continue five back blows and five chest thrusts until the object is dislodged or the infant loses consciousness. If the latter occurs, perform CPR. Each time you open the airway to deliver rescue breaths, look in the mouth and remove any object you see. Never perform a blind finger sweep.

Defibrillator paddle placement

Here's a guide to correct paddle placement for defibrillation.

Anterolateral placement

Place one paddle to the right of the upper sternum, just below the right clavicle, and the other over the fifth or sixth intercostal space at the left anterior axillary line.

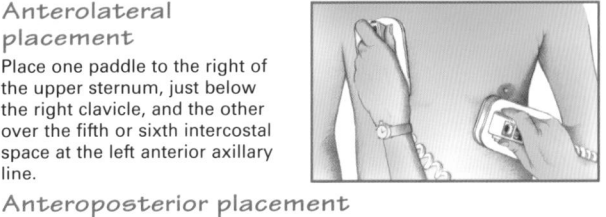

Anteroposterior placement

Place the anterior paddle directly over the heart at the precordium, to the left of the lower sternal border. Place the flat posterior paddle under the patient's body beneath the heart and immediately below the scapulae (but not under the vertebral column).

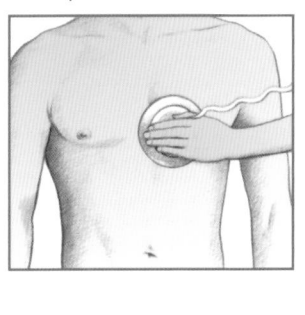
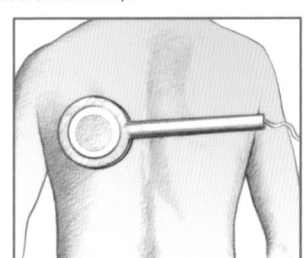

Choosing cardioversion energy level

When performing cardioversion, always start with the lowest energy level. For example:

• Unstable tachycardia with pulse or unstable atrial fibrillation with rapid ventricular response: 100 to 200 joules (monophasic) or 100 to 120 joules (biphasic). Increase the second and subsequent shock doses as needed.

• Unstable paroxysmal supraventricular tachycardia or unstable atrial flutter with rapid ventricular response: 50 to 100 joules (monophasic). Increase subsequent shock doses in a stepwise fashion.

Oxygen delivery

Oxygen delivery equipment	Oxygen concentration administered
Nasal cannula	1-6 L/min (24%-40% fraction of inspired oxygen [FIO_2])
Simple mask	5-8 L/min (40%-60% FIO_2)
Partial rebreather mask	6-15 L/min (40%-60% FIO_2)
Nonrebreather mask	6-15 L/min (55%-90% FIO_2)
Venturi mask	4-10 L/min (24%-55% FIO_2, depending on manufacturer)
Continuous positive airway pressure mask	Variable
Transtracheal oxygen	Variable
Aerosol mask	10-15 L/min
Handheld resuscitation bag (Ambu bag)	15 L/min

ACLS

The American Heart Association's ACLS course outlines specific protocols for treating life-threatening arrhythmias.

VF or pulseless VT

- CPR (stop when defibrillator ready)
- Defibrillate: 360 joules (monophasic) or 120 to 200 joules (biphasic)
- Resume CPR immediately
- Give 5 cycles of CPR and check rhythm
- Defibrillate: 360 joules (monophasic) or 120 to 200 joules (biphasic)
- Resume CPR
- Establish I.V. or I.O. access
- Epinephrine 1 mg I.V. or I.O. push q 3-5 min OR vasopressin 40 units I.V. × 1 only (to replace first or second dose of epinephrine)
- Give 5 cycles of CPR and check rhythm
- Defibrillate: 360 joules (monophasic) or 120 to 200 joules (biphasic)
- Resume CPR
- May consider:
  - amiodarone
  - lidocaine
  - magnesium sulfate
- Resume attempts to defibrillate

Pulseless electrical activity (PEA)

- CPR
- Establish I.V. or I.O. access
- Consider most common causes:
  5 H's:
  - Hypovolemia
  - Hypoxia
  - Hydrogen ion accumulation, resulting in acidosis
  - Hyperkalemia or hypokalemia
  - Hypothermia

5 T's:
- Tablets (accidental or deliberate drug overdose)
- Tamponade (cardiac)
- Tension pneumothorax
- Thrombosis (coronary)
- Thrombosis (pulmonary embolism)
- Epinephrine 1 mg I.V. or I.O. push q 3-5 min OR vasopressin 40 units I.V. or I.O. (to replace first or second dose of epinephrine)
- If PEA rate is slow (bradycardic), atropine 1 mg I.V. or I.O. q 3-5 min; maximum total dose 0.04 mg/kg
- Give 5 cycles of CPR and check rhythm

Asystole

- CPR
- Confirm true asystolic rhythm
- Establish I.V. or I.O. access
- Epinephrine 1 mg I.V. or I.O. push q 3-5 min OR vasopressin 40 units I.V. or I.O. (to replace first or second dose of epinephrine)
- Atropine 1 mg I.V. or I.O. q 3-5 min; maximum total dose 0.04 mg/kg
- Give 5 cycles of CPR and check rhythm
- Consider ceasing resuscitation if asystole persists

ACLS *(continued)*

Symptomatic bradycardia
- Ensure airway
- Oxygen
- Monitor ECG (identify rhythm)
- Establish I.V. access
- Vital signs, pulse oximetry
- If adequate perfusion, monitor patient
- If poor perfusion:
  - Transcutaneous pacing, if possible
  - Atropine 0.5 mg I.V.
  - Dopamine 2-10 mcg/kg/min
  - Epinephrine 2-10 mcg/min
  - Prepare for transvenous pacing
  - Treat contributing cause

Unstable, symptomatic tachycardia
- Ensure airway
- Oxygen
- Establish I.V. access
- Prepare for immediate cardioversion
- Premedicate whenever possible before cardioversion
- Synchronized cardioversion

Stable, monomorphic VT
- Ensure airway
- Oxygen
- Establish I.V. access
- Amiodarone 150 mg I.V. over 10 min. Repeat as needed to maximum dose of 2.2 g/24 hours.
- Synchronized cardioversion

Stable, narrow-complex supraventricular tachycardia with regular rhythm
- Ensure airway
- Oxygen
- Establish I.V. access
- Diagnosis: 12-lead ECG
- Treatment
  - vagal maneuvers
  - adenosine
- If rhythm doesn't convert:
  - control rate with antiarrhythmics
  - treat underlying cause

Stable, narrow-complex supraventricular tachycardia with irregular rhythm
- Ensure airway
- Oxygen
- Establish I.V. access
- Obtain 12-lead ECG
- Consider expert consultation
- Control rate with antiarrhythmics

Stable, wide-complex tachycardia with irregular rhythm
- Ensure airway
- Oxygen
- Establish I.V. access
- Seek expert consultation
- Consider antiarrhythmics

Rapid sequence intubation

Standard algorithm for adults

Preparation (< 10 min)

⬇

Pre-oxygenation (3-5 min or eight full vital capacity breaths of 100% oxygen)

⬇

Premedicate
a. *Sedate* (administer premedication — usually fentanyl, atropine [for children], lidocaine, etomidate, ketamine, midazolam, or thiopental — then wait 3 min after drug administration)
b. *Paralyze* (usually succinylcholine, rocuronium, vecuronium, atracurium, or pancuronium)
c. *Assess for apnea and jaw relaxation*

⬇

Protect airway
Perform cricoid pressure (Sellick maneuver) as soon as patient becomes unconscious and then wait 30 sec

⬇

Intubate (each attempt < 20 sec; max three attempts)
• If more than 1 attempt needed, ventilate patient for 30-60 sec with bag mask between attempts.
• After intubation, inflate balloon cuff.
• If patient becomes bradycardic during intubation, give atropine 0.5 mg I.V. push.

⬇

Verify tube placement (by clinical signs, end-tidal carbon dioxide using a capnometer, or esophageal device detector and by reconfirming that the ET tube actually passes between the cords by repeating direct laryngoscopy)

⬇

Post-tube management
• Secure ET tube.
• Set ventilator to appropriate settings.
• Continue administering sedative and muscle relaxant p.r.n.
• Obtain chest X-ray stat.
• Recheck vital signs and pulse oximetry.
• Perform continuous end-tidal capnometry (to detect accidental extubation).

Analyzing CO_2 levels

Disposable end-tidal carbon dioxide ($ETCO_2$) detectors are commonly used to confirm ET tube placement. The meaning of color changes within the detector dome differ depending on which detector you use. Here's a description of what color changes mean in the Easy Cap detector:

• The rim of the Easy Cap is divided into four segments (clockwise from the top): CHECK, A, B, and C. The CHECK segment is solid purple, signifying the absence of CO_2.

• The numbers in the other sections range from 0.03 to 5, indicating the percentage of exhaled CO_2. The color should fluctuate during ventilation from purple (section A) during inspiration to yellow (section C) at the end of expiration. This indicates that $ETCO_2$ levels are adequate (above 2%).

• An end-expiratory color change from C to the B range may be the first sign of hemodynamic instability.

• During CPR, an end-expiratory color change from the A or B range to the C range may mean the return of spontaneous ventilation.

• During prolonged cardiac arrest, inadequate pulmonary perfusion leads to inadequate gas exchange. The patient exhales little or no CO_2, so the color stays in the purple range even with proper intubation. Ineffective CPR also leads to inadequate pulmonary perfusion.

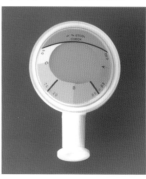

Troubleshooting ventilator alarms

Signal	Possible cause	Interventions
Low-pressure alarm	• Tube disconnection	• Reconnect tube to ventilator.
	• ET tube displaced	• Check tube placement; reposition, if needed. If extubation or displacement has occurred, ventilate patient manually. Call doctor immediately.
	• Leaking tidal volume from low cuff pressure	• Listen for whooshing sound around tube, indicating an air leak. If you hear one, check cuff pressure. If you can't maintain pressure, call doctor.
	• Ventilator malfunction	• Disconnect patient from ventilator and ventilate manually, if necessary. Obtain another ventilator.
	• Leak in ventilator circuitry	• Make sure all connections are intact. Check for holes or leaks in tubing. Check humidification jar and replace if cracked.
High-pressure alarm	• Increased airway pressure or decreased lung compliance	• Auscultate lungs for evidence of increasing lung consolidation, barotrauma, or wheezing. Call doctor if indicated.
	• Patient biting on oral ET tube	• Insert bite block if needed.
	• Secretions in airway	• Suction patient or have him cough.
	• Condensate in larger-bore tubing	• Check tubing for condensate and remove any fluid.
	• Intubation of right main stem bronchus	• Check tube position. If it has slipped, call doctor.
	• Patient coughing, gagging, or attempting to talk	• If patient fights the ventilator, doctor may order sedative or neuromuscular blocking agent.
	• Chest wall resistance	• Reposition patient to improve chest expansion. If repositioning doesn't help, administer prescribed analgesics.
	• Failure of high-pressure relief valve	• Replace faulty equipment.
	• Bronchospasm	• Assess for cause. Notify doctor.

Complications of mechanical ventilation and intubation

Mechanical ventilation

- Tension pneumothorax
- Decreased cardiac output
- Infection
- Volutrauma
- Organ impairment (renal, GI, CNS)

Intubation

- Trauma to teeth, lips, tongue
- Vocal cord injury
- Erosion of tracheal wall
- Ischemic pressure necrosis

Treating respiratory distress in mechanically ventilated patients

- Disconnect the ventilator from the ET or tracheostomy tube and manually ventilate with a handheld resuscitation bag at 100% oxygen.
- Check ventilator for problems. Alert respiratory therapy department.
- Assess the ET or tracheostomy tube for air leaks, and check cuff pressure. Notify the doctor if air leak is not corrected.
- Suction the ET or tracheostomy tube to clear secretions. Continue to ventilate manually.
- If the ET tube becomes dislodged, remove the tube and ventilate manually. Notify the doctor at once.
- If tracheostomy tube comes out, use a sterile tracheal dilator to keep the stoma open until a new tube can be inserted. Notify the doctor at once.

Arterial pressure monitoring

Normal arterial blood pressure produces a characteristic waveform representing ventricular systole and diastole. The waveform has five distinct components: the anacrotic limb, systolic peak, dicrotic limb, dicrotic notch, and end diastole.

The *anacrotic limb* marks the waveform's initial upstroke, which results as blood is rapidly ejected from the ventricle through the open aortic valve into the aorta. The rapid ejection causes a sharp rise in arterial pressure, which appears as the waveform's highest point. This is called the *systolic peak*.

As blood continues into the peripheral vessels, arterial pressure falls and the waveform begins a downward trend. This part is called the *dicrotic limb*. Arterial pressure usually continues to fall until pressure in the ventricle is less than pressure in the aortic root. When this occurs, the aortic valve closes. This event appears as a small notch on the waveform's downside, known as the *dicrotic notch*.

When the aortic valve closes, diastole begins, progressing until the aortic root pressure gradually descends to its lowest point. On the waveform, this is known as *end diastole*.

Normal arterial waveform

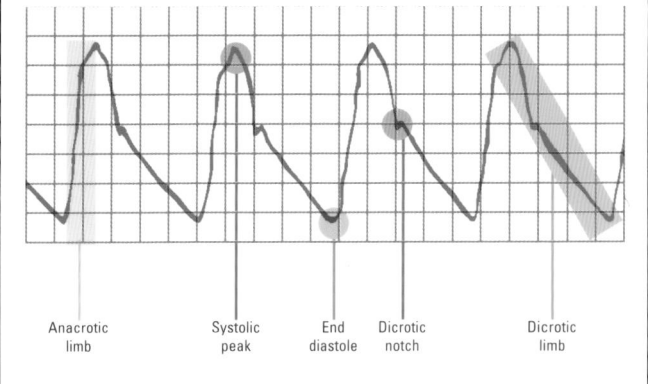

Anacrotic
limb

Systolic
peak

End
diastole

Dicrotic
notch

Dicrotic
limb

Normal PA waveforms

Right atrium

When the catheter tip enters the right atrium, a waveform like the one shown at right appears on the monitor. The *a* waves represent right ventricular end-diastolic pressure; the *v* waves, right atrial filling.

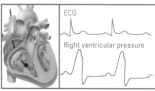

ECG

Right atrial pressure
a   v   a   v

Right ventricle

As the catheter tip reaches the right ventricle, you'll see a waveform with sharp systolic upstrokes and lower diastolic dips.

ECG

Right ventricular pressure

Pulmonary artery

The catheter then floats into the pulmonary artery, causing a waveform like the one shown at right. Note that the upstroke here is smoother than the one on the right ventricular waveform. The dicrotic notch indicates pulmonic valve closure.

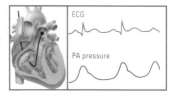

ECG

PA pressure

PAWP

Floating into a distal branch of the pulmonary artery, the balloon wedges where the vessel becomes too narrow for it to pass. The monitor now shows a PAWP waveform. The *a* waves represent left ventricular end-diastolic pressure; the *v* waves, left atrial filling.

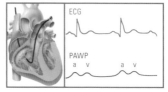

ECG

PAWP
a   v   a   v

Troubleshooting PA catheters

Problem	Possible causes	Interventions
No waveform	Transducer not open to catheter	• Check stopcock. • Reevaluate waveform.
	Transducer or monitor improperly set up	• Recheck all connections. • Rebalance transducer. • Replace system.
Overdamped waveform	Air in the line	• Check system for air. • Aspirate air.
	Clotted catheter tip	• Try to aspirate clot with a syringe according to facility policy. • If successful, flush line. • Don't try to flush line if clot can't be aspirated; notify doctor.
	Catheter tip lodged against vessel wall	• Reposition catheter according to facility policy. • Reposition patient. • Ask patient to cough.
Ventricular waveform tracing	Catheter migration into right ventricle	• Inflate balloon with 1.5 cc of air to move catheter into pulmonary artery. • If unsuccessful, notify doctor to reposition catheter.
Continuous PAWP waveform	Catheter migration or inflated balloon	• Reposition patient. • Ask patient to cough. • If unsuccessful, notify doctor.

Hemodynamic variables

Parameter and formula	Normal value
Mean arterial pressure (MAP) = $\dfrac{\text{Systolic blood pressure (BP)} + 2 \text{(diastolic BP)}}{3}$	70 to 105 mm Hg
Central venous pressure (CVP) or right atrial pressure (RAP)	2 to 6 cm H_2O; 2 to 8 mm Hg
Right ventricular pressure	20 to 30 mm Hg (systolic) 0 to 8 mm Hg (diastolic)
Pulmonary artery pressure (PAP)	20 to 30 mm Hg (systolic; PAS) 8 to 15 mm Hg (diastolic; PAD) 10 to 20 mm Hg (mean; PAM)
Pulmonary artery wedge pressure (PAWP)	4 to 12 mm Hg
Cardiac output (CO) = Heart rate (HR) $\times$ stroke volume (SV)	4 to 8 L/min
Cardiac index (CI) = $\dfrac{CO}{\text{Body surface area (BSA)}}$	2.5 to 4 L/min/m^2
Stroke volume (SV) = $\dfrac{CO}{HR}$	60 to 100 ml/beat
Stroke volume index = $\dfrac{SV}{BSA}$	30 to 60 ml/beat/m^2
Systemic vascular resistance = $\dfrac{MAP - RAP \times 80}{CO}$	900 to 1,200 dynes/sec/cm^{-5}
Systemic vascular resistance index = $\dfrac{MAP - RAP \times 80}{CI}$	1,360 to 2,200 dynes/sec/cm^{-5}/m^2

Transcutaneous pacemaker

Transcutaneous pacing involves the delivery of electrical impulses through externally applied cutaneous electrodes. The impulses are conducted through an intact chest wall using skin electrodes placed in either anterior-posterior (shown at right) or sternal-apex positions.

Transcutaneous pacing is the pacing method of choice in emergency situations because it's the least invasive technique and it can be instituted quickly.

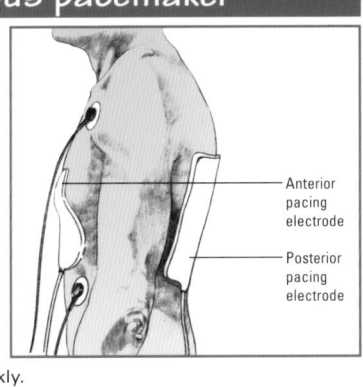

Anterior pacing electrode

Posterior pacing electrode

Understanding pacemaker codes

A permanent pacemaker's three-letter (or sometimes five-letter) code simply refers to how it's programmed.

First letter *(chamber that's paced)*	Second letter *(chamber that's sensed)*	Third letter *(pulse generator's response)*	Fourth letter *(pacemaker's programmability)*	Fifth letter *(pacemaker's response to tachycardia)*
A atrium	**A** atrium	**I** inhibited	**P** basic functions programmable	**P** pacing ability
V ventricle	**V** ventricle	**T** triggered	**M** multiple programmable parameters	**S** shock
D dual (both chambers)	**D** dual (both chambers)	**D** dual (inhibited and triggered)	**C** communicating functions such as telemetry	**D** dual ability to shock and pace
0 not applicable	**0** not applicable	**0** not applicable	**R** rate responsiveness	**0** none
			N none	

Positioning cardiac monitoring leads

Five-leadwire system	Three-leadwire system
Lead I 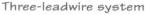	Lead I
Lead II	Lead II
Lead III	Lead III
Lead MCL₁	Lead MCL₁
Lead MCL₆	Lead MCL₆

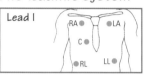

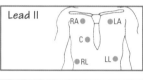

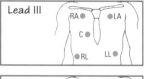

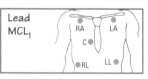

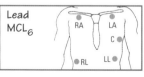

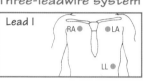

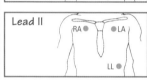

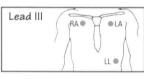

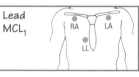

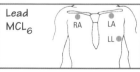

12-LEAD ECG

Precordial lead placement

To record the precordial chest leads, place the electrodes as follows:

V_1. . . . Fourth intercostal space (ICS), right sternal border
V_2. . . . Fourth ICS, left sternal border
V_3. . . . Midway between V_2 and V_4
V_4. . . . Fifth ICS, left midclavicular line
V_5. . . . Fifth ICS, left anterior axillary line
V_6. . . . Fifth ICS, left midaxillary line.

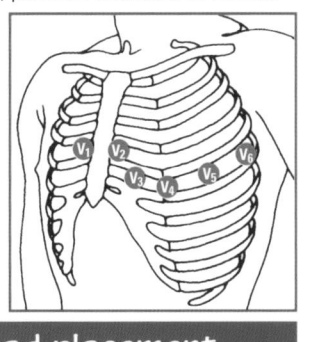

Right precordial lead placement

To record the right precordial chest leads, place the electrodes as follows:

V_1R . . Fourth intercostal space (ICS), left sternal-border
V_2R . . Fourth ICS, right sternal border
V_3R . . Halfway between V_2R and V_4R
V_4R . . Fifth ICS, right midclavicular line
V_5R . . Fifth ICS, right anterior axillary line
V_6R . . Fifth ICS, right midaxillary line

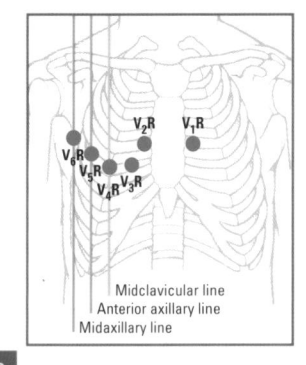

Midclavicular line
Anterior axillary line
Midaxillary line

Posterior lead placement

To ensure an accurate ECG reading, make sure the posterior electrodes V_7, V_8, and V_9 are placed at the same level horizontally as the V_6 lead at the fifth intercostal space. Place lead V_7 at the posterior axillary line, lead V_9 at the paraspinal line, and lead V_8 halfway between leads V_7 and V_9.

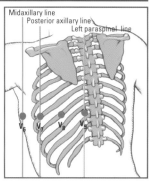

ECG grid

This ECG grid shows the horizontal axis and vertical axis and their respective measurement values.

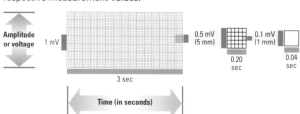

Normal sinus rhythm

Normal sinus rhythm, shown below, represents normal impulse conduction through the heart.

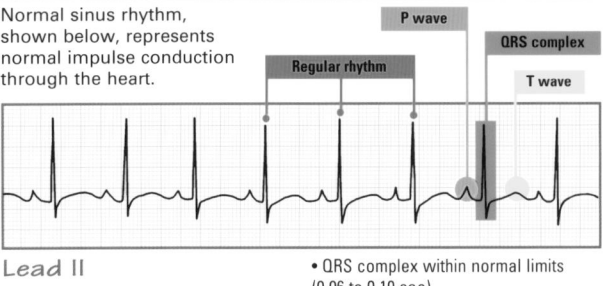

P wave

QRS complex

Regular rhythm

T wave

Lead II

- Atrial and ventricular rhythms regular
- Atrial and ventricular rates 60 to 100 beats/min (80 beats/min shown)
- Normal P wave preceding each QRS complex
- Normal PR interval (0.12 to 0.20 sec)

- QRS complex within normal limits (0.06 to 0.10 sec)
- T wave normally shaped (upright and rounded); follows each QRS complex
- QT interval within normal limits and constant (0.36 to 0.44 sec)

Sinus bradycardia

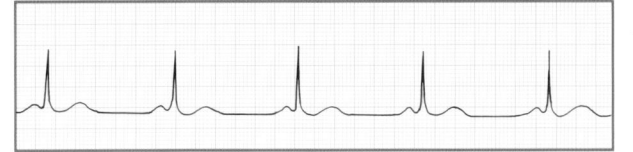

Rhythm . . . . regular
Rate . . . . < 60 beats/minute
P wave . . . . normal
PR interval . . . . . . 0.12 to 0.20 second
QRS complex . . . 0.06 to 0.10 second

Sinus tachycardia

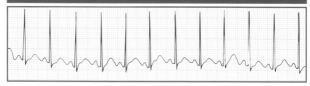

Rhythm . . . . regular
Rate . . . . 100 to 160 beats/minute
P wave . . . . normal
PR interval . . . . . . 0.12 to 0.20 second
QRS complex . . . 0.06 to 0.10 second

Premature atrial contractions (PACs)

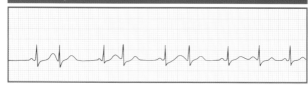

Rhythm . . . . irregular
Rate . . . . varies with underlying rhythm
P wave . . . . premature and abnormally shaped with premature atrial contractions
PR interval . . . . . . usually within normal limits, but varies depending on ectopic focus
QRS complex . . . 0.06 to 0.10 second

Atrial tachycardia

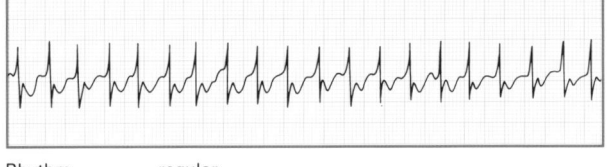

Rhythm . . . . regular
Rate . . . . 150 to 250 beats/minute; ventricular rate depends
                       on atrioventricular conduction rates
P wave . . . . hidden in the preceding T wave
PR interval . . . . . . not visible
QRS complex . . . 0.06 to 0.10 second

Atrial flutter

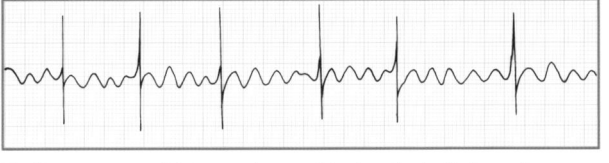

Rhythm . . . . atrial—regular; ventricular—typically irregular
Rate . . . . atrial—250 to 400 beats/minute;
                       ventricular—usually 60 to 100 beats/minute; ven-
                       tricular rate depends on degree of atrioventricular
                       block
P wave . . . . classic sawtooth appearance
PR interval . . . . . . unmeasurable
QRS complex . . . 0.06 to 0.10 second

Atrial fibrillation

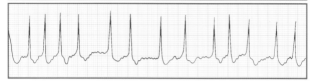

Rhythm . . . . irregularly irregular
Rate . . . . atrial—usually >400 beats/minute;
                       ventricular—varies
P wave . . . . absent; replaced by fine fibrillatory waves,
                       or f waves
PR interval . . . . . . indiscernible
QRS complex . . . 0.06 to 0.10 second

Premature junctional contractions (PJCs)

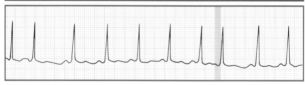

Rhythm . . . . irregular atrial and ventricular rhythms during
                       PJCs
Rate . . . . reflects the underlying rhythm
P wave . . . . usually inverted and may occur before or after or be
                       hidden within the QRS complex (see shaded area)
PR interval . . . . . . < 0.12 second if P wave precedes QRS complex;
                       otherwise unmeasurable
QRS complex . . . 0.06 to 0.10 second

Junctional escape rhythm

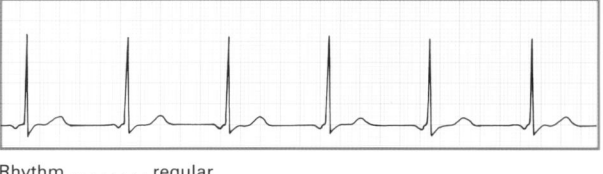

Rhythm . . . . regular
Rate . . . . 40 to 60 beats/minute
P wave. . . . . usually inverted and may occur before or after or be
hidden within QRS complex
PR interval. . . . . . < 0.12 second if P wave precedes QRS complex;
otherwise unmeasurable
QRS complex . . . 0.10 second

Accelerated junctional rhythm

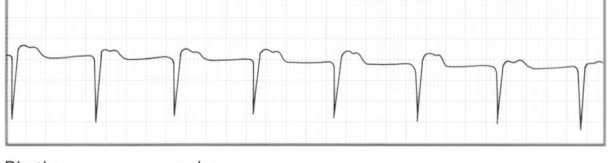

Rhythm . . . . regular
Rate . . . . 60 to 100 beats/minute
P wave. . . . . usually inverted and may occur before or after or be
hidden within QRS complex
PR interval. . . . . . < 0.12 second if P wave precedes QRS complex;
otherwise unmeasurable
QRS complex . . . 0.06 to 0.10 second

Premature ventricular contractions (PVCs)

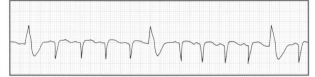

Rhythm . . . . irregular
Rate . . . . reflects the underlying rhythm
P wave . . . . none with PVC, but P wave present with other QRS
complexes
PR interval . . . . . . unmeasurable except in underlying rhythm
QRS complex . . . early, with bizarre configuration and duration of
> 0.12 second; QRS complexes are normal in under-
lying rhythm

Ventricular tachycardia

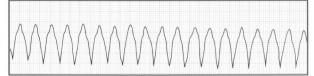

Rhythm . . . . regular
Rate . . . . atrial—can't be determined;
ventricular—100 to 250 beats/minute
P wave . . . . absent
PR interval . . . . . . unmeasurable
QRS complex . . . > 0.12 second; wide and bizarre

Ventricular fibrillation

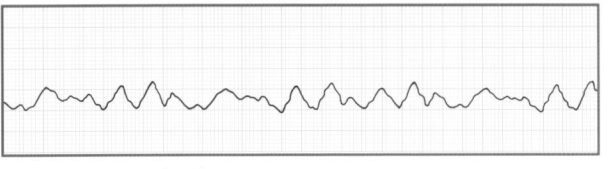

Rhythm . . . . chaotic
Rate . . . . can't be determined
P wave . . . . absent
PR interval . . . . . . unmeasurable
QRS complex . . . indiscernible

Asystole

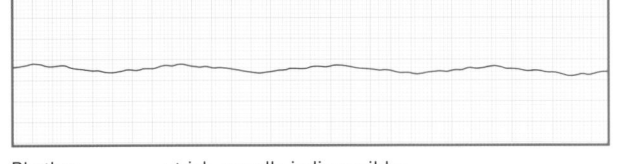

Rhythm . . . . atrial—usually indiscernible;
ventricular—absent
Rate . . . . atrial—usually indiscernible;
ventricular—absent
P wave . . . . may be present
PR interval . . . . . . unmeasurable
QRS complex . . . absent or occasional escape beats

First-degree atrioventricular block

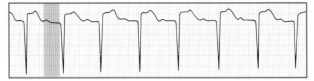

Rhythm . . . . regular
Rate . . . . within normal limits
P wave . . . . normal
PR interval . . . . . . > 0.20 second (see shaded area) but constant
QRS complex . . . 0.06 to 0.10 second

Type I second-degree atrioventricular block

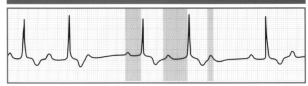

Rhythm . . . . atrial—regular; ventricular—irregular
Rate . . . . atrial—exceeds ventricular rate;
  both remain within normal limits
P wave . . . . normal
PR interval . . . . . . progressively prolonged (see shaded areas) until a
  P wave appears without a QRS complex
QRS complex . . . 0.06 to 0.10 second

Type II second-degree atrioventricular block

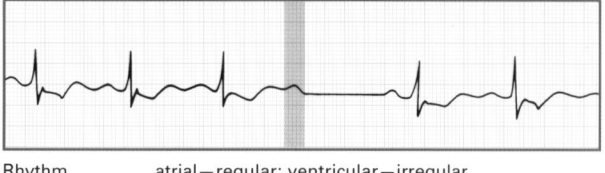

Rhythm . . . . atrial—regular; ventricular—irregular
Rate . . . . atrial—within normal limits; ventricular—slower
                    than atrial but may be within normal limits
P wave . . . . normal
PR interval . . . . . . constant for conducted beats
QRS complex . . . within normal limits; absent for dropped beats

Third-degree atrioventricular block

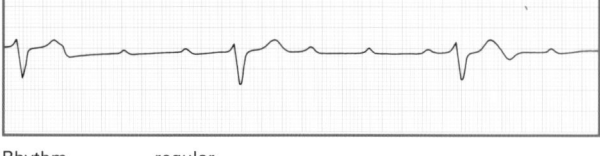

Rhythm . . . . regular
Rate . . . . atria and ventricles beat independently;
                    atrial—60 to 100 beats/minute;
                    ventricular—40 to 60 beats/minute intranodal block,
                    < 40 beats/minute infranodal block
P wave . . . . normal
PR interval . . . . . . varied; not applicable or measurable
QRS complex . . . normal or widened

Common dosage calculation formulas

$$\text{Body surface area in } m^2 = \sqrt{\frac{\text{height in cm} \times \text{weight in kg}}{3,600}}$$

$$\text{mcg/ml} = \text{mg/ml} \times 1,000$$

$$\text{ml/minute} = \frac{\text{ml/hour}}{60}$$

$$\text{gtt/minute} = \frac{\text{volume to be infused in ml}}{\text{time in minutes}} \times \text{drip factor in gtt/ml}$$

$$\text{mg/minute} = \frac{\text{mg in bag}}{\text{ml in bag}} \times \text{flow rate} \div 60$$

$$\text{mcg/minute} = \frac{\text{mg in bag}}{\text{ml in bag}} \div 0.06 \times \text{flow rate}$$

$$\text{mcg/kg/minute} = \frac{\text{mcg/ml} \times \text{ml/minute}}{\text{weight in kg}}$$

Calculating drip rates

When calculating the flow rate of I.V. solutions, remember that the number of drops required to deliver 1 ml varies with the type of administration set you're using. To calculate the drip rate, you must know the calibration of the drip rate for each specific manufacturer's product. As a quick guide, refer to the chart below. Use this formula to calculate specific drip rates:

$$\frac{\text{volume of infusion (in ml)}}{\text{time of infusion (in minutes)}} \times \text{drip factor (in drops/ml)} = \text{drops/minute}$$

	Ordered volume					
	500 ml/ 24 hr or 21 ml/hr	1,000 ml/ 24 hr or 42 ml/ hr	1,000 ml/ 20 hr or 50 ml/ hr	1,000 ml/ 10 hr or 100 ml/ hr	1,000 ml/ 8 hr or 125 ml/ hr	1,000 ml/6 hr or 166 ml/ hr
Drops/ml	**Drops/min to infuse**					
Macrodrip						
10	3	7	8	17	21	28
15	5	11	13	25	31	42
20	7	14	17	34	42	56
Microdrip						
60	21	42	50	100	125	166

Estimating BSA in children

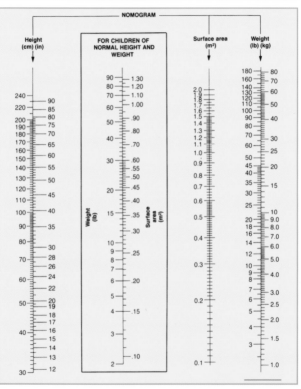

Adapted with permission from Behrman, R.E., et al. *Nelson Textbook of Pediatrics*, 16th ed. Philadelphia: W.B. Saunders Co., 1999.

Estimating BSA in adults

Height	Body surface area	Weight
cm 200 — 79 inch	2.80 m²	kg 150 — 330 lb
78	2.70	145 — 320
195 — 77	2.60	140 — 310
76	2.50	135 — 300
190 — 75	2.40	130 — 290
74		125 — 280
185 — 73	2.30	120 — 270
72	2.20	260
180 — 71	2.10	115 — 250
70		110 — 240
175 — 69	2.00	105 — 230
68	1.95	100 — 220
170 — 67	1.90	
66	1.85	95 — 210
165 — 65	1.80	90 — 200
64	1.75	85 — 190
160 — 63	1.70	80 — 180
62	1.65	
155 — 61	1.60	75 — 170
60	1.55	70 — 160
150 — 59	1.50	150
58	1.45	65 — 140
145 — 57	1.40	60 — 130
56	1.35	
140 — 55	1.30	55 — 120
54	1.25	
135 — 53	1.20	50 — 110
52	1.15	105
130 — 51	1.10	45 — 100
50	1.05	95
125 — 49	1.00	90
48	0.95	40 — 85
120 — 47	0.90	80
46	0.86 m²	35 — 75
115 — 45		70
44		
110 — 43		
42		
105 — 41		
40		
cm 100 — 39 in		kg 30 — 66 lb

Adapted with permission from *Geigy Scientific Tables,* 8th ed., 1990. Vol 5, p. 105.
© Novartis.

Determining compatibility for blood transfusions

		Compatible donors							
	(universal donor)	0−	0+	B−	B+	A−	A+	AB−	AB+
Patient's ABO group	(universal recipient) AB+	✔	✔	✔	✔	✔	✔	✔	✔
	AB−	✔		✔		✔		✔	
	A+	✔	✔			✔	✔		
	A−	✔				✔			
	B+	✔	✔	✔	✔				
	B−	✔		✔					
	0+	✔	✔						
	0−	✔							

I.V. solutions

Isotonic

Isotonic solutions expand the intravascular compartment. They include:
- D_5W
- 0.9% NaCl
- Ringer's injection
- lactated Ringer's injection.
  Monitor for fluid overload.

Hypertonic

Hypertonic solutions greatly expand the intravascular compartment and draw fluid from intravascular areas. They include:
- $D_{10}W$
- 3% NaCl
- 5% NaCl
- D_5LR
- $D_5$0.45% NaCl
- $D_5$0.9% NaCl.
  Monitor for fluid overload.

Hypotonic

Hypotonic solutions cause a fluid shift from the intravascular compartment into the cells. They include:
- $D_{2.5}W$
- 0.45% NaCl
- 0.33% NaCl.
  Monitor for cardiovascular collapse.

Common antidotes

Drug or toxin	Antidote
Acetaminophen	Acetylcysteine (Mucomyst)
Anticholinergics	Physostigmine (Antilirium)
Benzodiazepines	Flumazenil (Romazicon)
Calcium channel blockers	Calcium chloride
Cyanide	Amyl nitrate, sodium nitrite, and sodium thio-sulfate (Cyanide Antidote Kit); methylene blue
Digoxin, cardiac glycosides	Digoxin immune Fab (Digibind)
Ethylene glycol	Ethanol
Heparin	Protamine sulfate
Insulin-induced hypoglycemia	Glucagon
Iron	Deferoxamine mesylate (Desferal)
Lead	Edetate calcium disodium (Calcium Disodium Versenate)
Opioids	Naloxone (Narcan), nalmefene (Revex), naltrexone (ReVia)
Organophosphates, anticholinesterases	Atropine, pralidoxime (Protopam)
Warfarin	Vitamin K

Therapeutic drug monitoring

Drug	Laboratory test	Therapeutic range
Digoxin	Digoxin	0.8-2 mg/ml (SI: 1.0-2.6 mmol/L)
Phenytoin	Phenytoin	10-20 mcg/ml (SI: 40-79 µmol/L)
Procainamide	Procainamide	4-10 mcg/ml (SI: 17-42 µmol/L)
	N-acetylprocainamide (NAPA)	5-30 mcg/ml (combined pro-cainamide and NAPA)
Theophylline	Theophylline	10-20 mcg/ml (SI: 44-111 µmol/L)

Epinephrine and isoproterenol

Epinephrine

Mix 1 mg in 250 ml (4 mcg/ml) of D_5W.

Dose (mcg/min)	Infusion rate (ml/hr)
1	15
2	30
3	45
4	60
5	75
6	90
7	105
8	120
9	135
10	150
15	225
20	300
25	375
30	450
35	525
40	600

Isoproterenol

Mix 1 mg in 250 ml (4 mcg/ml) of D_5W.

Dose (mcg/min)	Infusion rate (ml/hr)
0.5	8
1	15
2	30
3	45
4	60
5	75
6	90
7	105
8	120
9	135
10	150
15	225
20	300
25	375
30	450

Nitroglycerin

Determine the infusion rate in ml/hr using the ordered dose and the concentration of the drug solution.

Dose (mcg/min)	25 mg/250 ml (100 mcg/ml)	50 mg/250 ml (200 mcg/ml)	100 mg/250 ml (400 mcg/ml)
5	3	2	1
10	6	3	2
20	12	6	3
30	18	9	5
40	24	12	6
50	30	15	8
60	36	18	9
70	42	21	10
80	48	24	12
90	54	27	14
100	60	30	15
150	90	45	23
200	120	60	30

Dobutamine

Mix 250 mg in 250 ml of D$_5$W (1,000 mcg/ml). Determine the infusion rate in ml/hr, using the ordered dose and the patient's weight in pounds or kilograms.

Dose (mcg/kg/min)	Patient's weight														
lb	88	99	110	121	132	143	154	165	176	187	198	209	220	231	242
kg	40	45	50	55	60	65	70	75	80	85	90	95	100	105	110
2.5	6	7	8	8	9	10	11	11	12	13	14	14	15	16	17
5	12	14	15	17	18	20	21	23	24	26	27	29	30	32	33
7.5	18	20	23	25	27	29	32	34	36	38	41	43	45	47	50
10	24	27	30	33	36	39	42	45	48	51	54	57	60	63	66
12.5	30	34	38	41	45	49	53	56	60	64	68	71	75	79	83
15	36	41	45	50	54	59	63	68	72	77	81	86	90	95	99
20	48	54	60	66	72	78	84	90	96	102	108	114	120	126	132
25	60	68	75	83	90	98	105	113	120	128	135	143	150	158	165
30	72	81	90	99	108	117	126	135	144	153	162	171	180	189	198
35	84	95	105	116	126	137	147	158	168	179	189	200	210	221	231
40	96	108	120	132	144	156	168	180	192	204	216	228	240	252	264

Dopamine

Mix 400 mg in 250 ml of D$_5$W (1,600 mcg/ml). Determine the infusion rate in ml/hr, using the ordered dose and the patient's weight in pounds or kilograms.

Patient's weight

Dose (mcg/kg/min)	lb 88 kg 40	99 45	110 50	121 55	132 60	143 65	154 70	165 75	176 80	187 85	198 90	209 95	220 100	231 105
2.5	4	4	5	5	6	6	7	7	8	8	8	9	9	10
5	8	8	9	10	11	12	13	14	15	16	17	18	19	20
7.5	11	13	14	15	17	18	20	21	23	24	25	27	28	30
10	15	17	19	21	23	24	26	28	30	32	34	36	38	39
12.5	19	21	23	26	28	30	33	35	38	40	42	45	47	49
15	23	25	28	31	34	37	39	42	45	48	51	53	56	59
20	30	34	38	41	45	49	53	56	60	64	68	71	75	79
25	38	42	47	52	56	61	66	70	75	80	84	89	94	98
30	45	51	56	62	67	73	79	84	90	96	101	107	113	118
35	53	59	66	72	79	85	92	98	105	112	118	125	131	138
40	60	68	75	83	90	98	105	113	120	128	135	143	150	158
45	68	76	84	93	101	110	118	127	135	143	152	160	169	177
50	75	84	94	103	113	122	131	141	150	159	169	178	188	197

Nitroprusside

Mix 50 mg in 250 ml of D_5W (200 mcg/ml). Determine the infusion rate in ml/hr, using the ordered dose and the patient's weight in pounds or kilograms.

Dose (mcg/kg/min)	lb 88 kg 40	99 45	110 50	121 55	132 60	143 65	154 70	165 75	176 80	187 85	198 90	209 95	220 100	231 105	242 110
							Patient's weight								
0.3	4	4	5	5	5	6	6	7	7	8	8	9	9	9	10
0.5	6	7	8	8	9	10	11	11	12	13	14	14	15	16	17
1	12	14	15	17	18	20	21	23	24	26	27	29	30	32	33
1.5	18	20	23	25	27	29	32	34	36	38	41	43	45	47	50
2	24	27	30	33	36	39	42	45	48	51	54	57	60	63	66
3	36	41	45	50	54	59	63	68	72	77	81	86	90	95	99
4	48	54	60	66	72	78	84	90	96	102	108	114	120	126	132
5	60	68	75	83	90	98	105	113	120	128	135	143	150	158	165
6	72	81	90	99	108	117	126	135	144	153	162	171	180	189	198
7	84	95	105	116	126	137	147	158	168	179	189	200	210	221	231
8	96	108	120	132	144	156	168	180	192	204	216	228	240	252	264
9	108	122	135	149	162	176	189	203	216	230	243	257	270	284	297
10	120	135	150	165	180	195	210	225	240	255	270	285	300	315	330

BURNS

Causes of burns

Type	Causes
Thermal	Flames, radiation, or excessive heat from fire, steam, or hot liquids or objects
Chemical	Various acids, bases, and caustics
Electrical	Electrical current and lightning
Light	Intense light sources or ultraviolet light, including sunlight
Radiation	Nuclear radiation and ultraviolet light

Classifying burns

Burns are classified according to the depth of the injury, as follows:
• **First-degree burns** are limited to the epidermis. Sunburn is a typical first-degree burn. These burns are painful but self-limiting. They don't lead to scarring and require only local wound care.
• **Second-degree burns** extend into the dermis but leave some residual dermis viable. These burns are painful and the skin will appear swollen and red with blister formation.
• **Third-degree,** or **full-thickness, burns** involve destruction of the entire dermis, leaving only S.C. tissue exposed. These burns look dry and leathery and are painless because the nerve endings are destroyed.
• **Fourth-degree burns** are a rare type of burn usually associated with lethal injury. They extend beyond the S.C. tissue, involving the muscle, fasciae, and bone. Occasionally termed *transmural burns,* these injuries are commonly associated with complete transection of an extremity.

Estimating the extent of burns

Rule of Nines

Use to estimate the extent of an adult patient's burns.

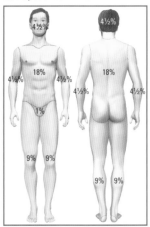

Lund and Browder chart

Use to estimate the extent of an infant's or a child's burns.

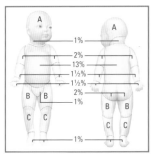

Relative percentages of areas affected by age

	At birth	0 to 1 yr	1 to 4 yr	5 to 9 yr	10 to 15 yr	Adult
A: Half of head						
	9½%	8½%	6½%	5½%	4½%	3½%
B: Half of thigh						
	2½%	3½%	4%	4½%	4½%	4½%
C: Half of leg						
	2½%	2½%	2½%	3%	3½%	3½%

Comparing types of chest pain

What it feels like	Where it's located	What makes it better	What makes it worse	What causes it
Aching, squeezing, burning pain as well as pressure and heaviness; usually subsides within 10 minutes	Substernal; may radiate to jaw, neck, arms, or back	Rest, nitroglycerin (*Note:* Unstable angina appears even at rest.)	Eating, physical effort, smoking, cold weather, stress, anger, hunger, lying down	Angina pectoris
Tightness or pressure; burning, aching pain, possibly accompanied by shortness of breath, diaphoresis, weakness, anxiety, or nausea; sudden onset; lasts 30 minutes to 2 hours	Typically across chest but may radiate to jaw, neck, arms, or back	Opioid analgesics, such as morphine and nitroglycerin	Exertion, anxiety	Acute MI
Sharp and continuous; may be accompanied by friction rub; sudden onset	Substernal; may radiate to neck or left arm	Sitting up, leaning forward, anti-inflammatory drugs	Deep breathing, supine position	Pericarditis
Excruciating, tearing pain; may be accompanied by blood pressure difference between right and left arm; sudden onset	Retrosternal, upper abdominal, or epigastric; may radiate to back, neck, or shoulders	Analgesics, surgery	Not applicable	Dissecting aortic aneurysm

(continued)

Comparing types of chest pain (continued)

What it feels like	Where it's located	What makes it better	What makes it worse	What causes it
Sudden, stabbing pain; possibly cyanosis, dyspnea, or cough with hemoptysis	Over lung area	Analgesics	Inspiration	Pulmonary embolus
Sudden, severe pain; may experience dyspnea, increased pulse rate, decreased breath sounds, or deviated trachea	Lateral thorax	Analgesics, chest tube insertion	Normal respiration	Pneumothorax

Comparing types of abdominal pain

Description	Location	Possible causes
Visceral: Originates in an abdominal organ; caused by stretching of nerve fibers around the organ; may be cramping, gaslike, colicky, intermittent; may vary in intensity	Periumbilical	Appendicitis, cholecystitis, gastroenteritis, bowel obstruction, renal colic
Parietal or somatic: Caused by chemical or bacterial irritation; often rapid onset; sharp, steady, and severe in intensity	Localized	Viral or bacterial peritonitis, late appendicitis, gastroenteritis
Referred: Caused by irritation of shared dermatomes of affected organ	Distant from site of pathology	MI, angina, pancreatitis, renal colic, abdominal aortic aneurysm

Classifying fractures

General classification

- Simple (closed)—Bone fragments don't penetrate the skin.
- Compound (open)—Bone fragments penetrate the skin.
- Incomplete (partial)—Bone continuity isn't completely interrupted.
- Complete—Bone continuity is completely interrupted.

By fragment position

- Comminuted—Bone breaks into small pieces.
- Impacted—One bone fragment is forced into another.
- Angulated—Fragments lie at an angle to each other.
- Displaced—Fragments separate and are deformed.
- Nondisplaced—Two sections of bone maintain essentially normal alignment.
- Overriding—Fragments overlap, shortening the total bone length.
- Segmental—Fractures occur in two adjacent areas with an isolated central segment.
- Avulsed—Fragments are pulled from the normal position by muscle contractions or ligament resistance.

By fracture line

- Linear—Fracture line runs parallel to the bone's axis.

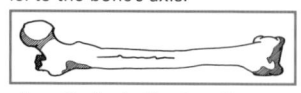

- Longitudinal—Fracture line extends in a longitudinal (but not parallel) direction along the bone's axis.

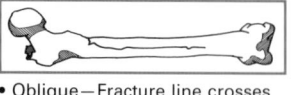

- Oblique—Fracture line crosses the bone at about a 45-degree angle to the bone's axis.

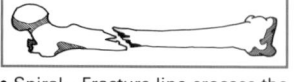

- Spiral—Fracture line crosses the bone at an oblique angle, creating a spiral pattern.

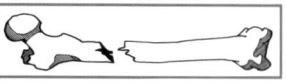

- Transverse—Fracture line forms a right angle with the bone's axis.

Managing fractures in the ED

Expose — Expose the site by removing all clothing and jewelry near the suspected fracture.

Physical assessment — Inspect for color, position, disrupted skin, bleeding, deformity, and differences compared with the uninjured side. Assess the extremity for pain, pallor, pulses, paresthesia, and paralysis (five P's).

When to splint — Splint for deformity, pain, bony crepitus, edema, ecchymosis, vascular compromise, open wounds, paralysis, and paresthesia.

Immobilize — Use a splint that effectively immobilizes the joints below and above the injury. Avoid manipulating the bone.
• Rigid splints (plastic and metal) are used for lower extremity fractures.
• Soft splints, such as pillows and slings, are used for upper extremity fractures.
• Traction splints are used for femur and proximal tibial fractures.

PRICE — This mnemonic reminds you to **p**rotect, **r**est, apply **i**ce, **c**ompress, and **e**levate the site. Ice and elevation are essential ED procedures.

Medications — Administer analgesics.

Diagnostic testing — Order X-rays. The views should include the joints above and below the injury.

Ongoing monitoring — Frequently reassess the five P's: pain, pallor, pulses, paresthesia, and paralysis.

Anticipate — Anticipate definitive stabilization, traction, internal or external fixation, and hospitalization for closed or open reduction.

Types of head trauma

Type	Description

Concussion (closed head injury)	• A blow to the head hard enough to make the brain hit the skull but not hard enough to cause a cerebral contusion; causes temporary neural dysfunction
	• Signs and symptoms:
	  – Short-term loss of consciousness
	  – Irritability or lethargy
	  – Dizziness, nausea, vomiting, or severe headache

Contusion (bruising of brain tissue; more serious than concussion)	• Blood accumulates between skull and dura (commonly from arterial bleeding).
	• Signs and symptoms:
	  – Severe scalp wounds
	  – Labored respiration and loss of consciousness
	  – Drowsiness, confusion, disorientation, agitation, or violent behavior (from increased ICP)
	  – Hemiparesis
	  – Decorticate or decerebrate posturing
	  – Unequal pupillary response

Epidural hematoma	• Injury occurs directly beneath the site of impact when the brain rebounds against the skull from the force of a blow.
	• Signs and symptoms:
	  – Brief period of unconsciousness after injury (reflecting concussive effects of head trauma), followed by a lucid interval of 10 minutes to hours or, rarely, days
	  – Severe headache
	  – Progressive loss of consciousness and deterioration of neurologic status
	  – Respirations initially deep and labored, becoming shallow and irregular
	  – Contralateral motor deficits
	  – Ipsilateral (same-side) pupillary dilation
	  – Seizures possible from increased ICP
	  – Continued bleeding leading to progressive neurologic degeneration

Types of head trauma *(continued)*

Type	Description
Subdural hematoma	• Meningeal hemorrhages resulting from accumulation of blood in subdural space • Signs and symptoms: – Similar to epidural hematoma but significantly slower onset
Intracerebral hematoma	• Traumatic or spontaneous disruption of cerebral vessels in brain parenchyma cause neurologic deficits, depending on site and amount of bleeding. • Signs and symptoms: – Unresponsive immediately or lucid before lapsing into a coma from increasing ICP and hemorrhage – Possible motor deficits and decorticate or decerebrate posture
Skull fractures	• Four types: linear, comminuted, depressed, and basilar • Signs and symptoms: – Possibly asymptomatic, depending on underlying brain trauma – Motor, sensory, and cranial nerve dysfunction associated with facial fractures – Periorbital ecchymosis (raccoon eyes), anosmia (loss of smell due to first cranial nerve involvement), and pupil abnormalities (due to second and third cranial nerve involvement) possible with anterior fossa basilar skull fractures – CSF rhinorrhea (leakage through nose), CSF otorrhea (leakage from ear), hemotympanum (blood accumulation at tympanic membrane), ecchymosis over mastoid bone (Battle's sign), and facial paralysis with middle fossa basilar skull fractures – Signs of medullary dysfunction, such as cardiovascular and respiratory failure, with posterior fossa basilar skull fractures

Managing heart failure

The New York Heart Association (NYHA) classification of heart failure is based on functional capacity. The American College of Cardiology/American Heart Association (ACC/AHA) guidelines are based on objective assessment.

NYHA classification	ACC/AHA guidelines	Recommendations
—	**Stage A:** High risk of developing HF without structural heart disease or signs and symptoms of HF	• Treatment of hypertension, lipid disorders, and diabetes • Smoking cessation and regular exercise • Discouraging use of alcohol and illicit drugs • ACE inhibitor
Class I: Ordinary physical activity doesn't cause undue fatigue, palpitations, dyspnea, or angina.	**Stage B:** Structural heart disease without signs and symptoms of HF	• All stage A therapies • ACE inhibitor (unless contraindicated) • Beta-adrenergic blocker (unless contraindicated)

(continued)

Managing heart failure (continued)

NYHA classification	ACC/AHA guidelines	Recommendations
Class II: Slight limitation of physical activity but asymptomatic at rest. Ordinary physical activity causes fatigue, palpitations, dyspnea, or angina. **Class III:** Marked limitation of physical activity but typically asymptomatic at rest. Less than ordinary physical activity causes fatigue, palpitations, dyspnea, or angina.	**Stage C:** Structural heart disease with prior or current signs and symptoms of HF	• All stage A and B therapies • Sodium-restricted diet • Avoiding or withdrawing antiarrhythmics, most calcium channel blockers, and NSAIDs • Drug therapy, including diuretics, digoxin, aldosterone antagonists, angiotensin receptor blockers, hydralazine, and nitrates
Class IV: Unable to perform any physical activity without discomfort; symptoms may be present even at rest. Discomfort increases with physical activity.	**Stage D:** End-stage disease requiring specialized treatments, such as mechanical circulatory support, continuous inotropic infusion, or heart transplantation	• All therapies for stages A, B, and C • Mechanical assist device, such as biventricular pacemaker or left ventricular assist device • Continuous inotropic therapy • Hospice care

ER Care

Types of seizures

Type	Description	Signs and symptoms
Partial		
Simple partial	Symptoms confined to one hemisphere	Possibly motor (change in posture), sensory (hallucinations), or autonomic (flushing, tachycardia) symptoms; no loss of consciousness
Complex partial	Begins in one focal area, but spreads to both hemispheres (more common in adults)	Loss of consciousness; aura of visual disturbances; postictal symptoms (such as amnesia, drowsiness, weakness)
Generalized		
Absence (petit mal)	Sudden onset; lasts 5 to 10 seconds; can have 100 daily; precipitated by stress, hyperventilation, hypoglycemia, fatigue; differentiated from daydreaming	Loss of responsiveness, but continued ability to maintain posture control and not fall; twitching eyelids; lip smacking; no postictal symptoms
Clonic	Muscles contract and relax in rhythmic pattern; may occur in one limb more than others	Mucus production
Tonic	Continuous contracted state (rigid posture)	Variable loss of consciousness; pupils dilate and eyes roll up; glottis closes; possibly incontinence and foaming at mouth
Tonic-clonic (grand mal, major motor)	Violent total body seizure	Aura; tonic first (20 to 40 seconds), then clonic; postictal symptoms
Atonic	Drop and fall attack	Loss of posture control
Akinetic	Sudden, brief loss of muscle tone or posture	Temporary loss of consciousness

(continued)

Types of seizures (continued)

Type	Description	Signs and symptoms
Unclassified		
Febrile	Seizure threshold lowered by elevated temperature; only one seizure per fever; occurs when temperature is rapidly rising	Lasts less than 5 minutes; generalized, transient, and nonprogressive; doesn't usually result in brain damage; EEG is normal after 2 weeks
Status epilepticus	Prolonged or frequent repetition of seizures without interruption; results in anoxia and cardiac and respiratory arrest	Consciousness not regained between seizures; lasts more than 30 minutes

Status epilepticus

Status epilepticus is a continuous seizure state that must be interrupted by emergency measures. It can occur during all types of seizures. For example, generalized tonic-clonic status epilepticus is a continuous generalized tonic-clonic seizure without an intervening return of consciousness.

Always an emergency

Status epilepticus is accompanied by respiratory distress. It can result from withdrawal of antiepileptic drugs, hypoxic or metabolic encephalopathy, acute head trauma, or septicemia secondary to encephalitis or meningitis.

Act fast

Emergency treatment usually consists of diazepam, phenytoin, or phenobarbital; I.V. dextrose 50% when seizures are secondary to hypoglycemia; and I.V. thiamine for patients with chronic alcoholism or those who are undergoing withdrawal.

Types of spinal cord injury

Type	Description	Signs and symptoms
Complete transection	• All spinal cord tracts completely disrupted • All functions involving spinal cord below level of transection lost • Complete and permanent loss	• Loss of motor function (quadriplegia) with cervical cord transection; paraplegia with thoracic cord transection • Muscle flaccidity • Loss of all reflexes and sensory function below level of injury • Bladder and bowel atony; paralytic ileus • Loss of vasomotor tone in lower body parts with low and unstable blood pressure • Loss of perspiration below level of injury • Pale, dry skin • Respiratory impairment
Incomplete transection: central cord syndrome	• Center portion of cord affected • Typically results from hyper-extension injury	• More motor deficits in upper extremities than in lower extremities • Variable degree of bladder dysfunction
Incomplete transection: anterior cord syndrome	• Occlusion of anterior spinal artery from pressure of bone fragments	• Loss of motor function below level of injury • Loss of pain and temperature sensations below level of injury • Intact touch, pressure, position, and vibration senses
Incomplete transection: Brown-Séquard syndrome	• Hemisection of cord affected • Most common in stabbing and gunshot wounds • Damage to cord on one side	• Ipsilateral paralysis or paresis below level of injury • Ipsilateral loss of touch, pressure, vibration, and position senses below level of injury • Contralateral loss of pain and temperature sensations below level of injury

Managing shock

Types	Pathophysiology	Causes	Physical findings	Treatment
Anaphylactic	• Edema • Blood vessel dilation • Bronchospasms • Fluid shifts	• Allergic reaction to antigens	• Pale, cool skin • Hypotension • Respiratory distress • Edema • Rash	• Epinephrine • Corticosteroids • Antihistamines • I.V. fluids • Oxygen
Cardiogenic	• Decreased cardiac output • Left ventricular dysfunction • Sympathetic compensation • Myocardial ischemia	• MI • Myocardial ischemia • Myocarditis • Papillary muscle dysfunction • Ventricular septal defect • Ventricular aneurysm • Acute mitral or aortic insufficiency	• Pale, cool, clammy skin • Decreased sensorium • Rapid, thready pulse • Rapid, shallow respirations • Mean arterial pressure < 60 mm Hg in adults • Gallop rhythm • Faint heart sounds	• Vasopressors • Inotropics • Vasoconstrictors • Osmotic diuretics • Oxygen • IABP • Analgesics, sedatives

(continued)

Managing shock *(continued)*

Types	Pathophysiology	Causes	Physical findings	Treatment
Hypovolemic	• Reduced venous return to heart due to lost fluid • Decreased ventricular filling • Decreased cardiac output • Tissue anoxia • Metabolic acidosis	• Acute blood loss • Intestinal obstruction • Burns • Peritonitis • Acute pancreatitis • Ascites • Dehydration	• Pale, cool, clammy skin • Decreased sensorium • Rapid, shallow respirations • Urine output < 20 ml/hr • Rapid, thready pulse • Mean arterial pressure < 60 mm Hg in adults • Orthostatic vital signs	• Prompt, vigorous blood and fluid replacement • Positive inotropics • Possible diuretics
Neurogenic	• Severe vasodilation	• Anesthesia • Spinal cord injury	• Pale, warm, dry skin • Bounding pulse • Bradycardia • Hypotension	• I.V. fluids • Oxygen • Vasopressors • Lying flat
Septic	• Activation of chemical mediators in response to invading organisms • Functional hypovolemia	• Any pathogenic organism • Primarily gram-negative bacteria	*Early* • Pink, flushed skin • Rapid, shallow respirations • Rapid, full, bounding pulse • Normal or slightly elevated blood pressure *Late* • Pale, cyanotic skin • Rapid, shallow respirations • Rapid, weak, thready pulse • Hypotension	• Antimicrobials • Colloids or crystalloids • Oxygen • Diuretics • Vasopressors

Locating myocardial damage

After you've noted characteristic lead changes in an acute MI, use this table to identify the areas of damage. Match the lead changes (ST elevation, abnormal Q waves) in the second column with the affected wall in the first column and the artery involved in the third column. The fourth column shows reciprocal lead changes.

Wall affected	Leads	Artery involved	Reciprocal changes
Anterior	V_2, V_3, V_4	Left coronary artery, left anterior descending (LAD)	II, III, aV_F
Anterolateral	I, aV_L, V_3, V_4, V_5, V_6	LAD and diagonal branches, circumflex and marginal branches	II, III, aV_F
Anteroseptal	V_1, V_2, V_3, V_4	LAD	None
Inferior	II, III, aV_F	Right coronary artery (RCA)	I, aV_L
Lateral	I, aV_L, V_5, V_6	Circumflex branch of left coronary artery	II, III, aV_F
Posterior	V_8, V_9	RCA or circumflex	V_1, V_2, V_3, V_4 (R greater than S in V_1 and V_2, ST-segment depression, elevated T wave)
Right ventricular	V_{4R}, V_{5R}, V_{6R}	RCA	None

Stroke signs and symptoms

Site	Signs and symptoms
Middle cerebral artery	• Aphasia • Dysphasia • Dyslexia • Dysgraphia • Visual field cuts • Hemiparesis on affected side; more severe in face and arm than in leg
Internal carotid artery	• Headache • Weakness • Paralysis • Numbness • Sensory changes • Visual disturbances, such as blurring on affected side • Altered level of consciousness • Bruits over the carotid artery • Aphasia • Dysphagia • Ptosis
Posterior cerebral artery	• Visual field cuts • Sensory impairment • Dyslexia • Coma • Blindness from ischemia in occipital area

Site	Signs and symptoms
Anterior cerebral artery	• Confusion • Weakness • Numbness on affected side (especially in arm) • Paralysis of contralateral foot and leg • Incontinence • Poor coordination • Impaired motor and sensory function • Personality changes, such as flat affect and distractibility
Vertebral or basilar artery	• Mouth and lip numbness • Dizziness • Weakness on affected side • Visual deficits, such as color blindness, lack of depth perception, and diplopia • Poor coordination • Dysphagia • Slurred speech • Amnesia • Ataxia

Criteria for thrombolytic therapy

Evaluate every stroke patient prior to administering thrombolytic therapy to determine whether established criteria are met.

Criteria that must be present

- Age 18 years or older
- Acute ischemic stroke associated with significant neurologic deficit
- Symptom onset < 3 hours before treatment begins

Criteria that must not be present

- Evidence of intracranial hemorrhage during pretreatment evaluation
- Evidence of subarachnoid hemorrhage during pretreatment evaluation
- Evidence of multilobar infarction on CT scan
- History of recent (within 3 months) intracranial or intraspinal surgery, serious head trauma, or previous stroke
- History of intracranial hemorrhage
- Uncontrolled hypertension at time of treatment
- Seizure at onset of stroke
- Active internal bleeding or acute trauma
- Intracranial neoplasm, arteriovenous malformation, or aneurysm
- Known bleeding diathesis involving, but not limited to:
  – current use of oral anticoagulants, such as warfarin, with elevated INR or PT
  – International Normalized Ratio > 1.7
  – PT > 15 seconds
  – receipt of heparin within 48 hours before onset of stroke and elevated PTT
  – platelet count < 100,000/µl
- Arterial puncture at a noncompressible site (within 7 days)

Whiplash injuries

Whiplash injuries result from sharp hyperextension and hyperflexion of the neck that damages muscles, ligaments, disks, and nerve tissue. The prognosis is usually excellent after treatment of symptoms.

Causes

- Motor vehicle accidents
- Falls
- Sports-related accidents
- Crimes and assaults

Signs and symptoms

Although symptoms may develop immediately, they're often delayed 12 to 24 hours if the injury is mild. Whiplash produces moderate to severe anterior and posterior neck pain. Within several days, the anterior pain diminishes, but the posterior pain persists or even intensifies, causing patients to seek medical attention if they did not do so before.

Whiplash may also cause:
- dizziness
- gait disturbances
- vomiting
- headache
- nuchal rigidity
- neck muscle asymmetry
- rigidity or numbness in the arms.

Treatment

- Immobilization with a soft, padded cervical collar for several days or weeks
- Ice or cool compresses to the neck
- Mild analgesic and possibly a muscle relaxant
- For severe muscle spasms, short-term cervical traction

Hyperflexion Hyperextension

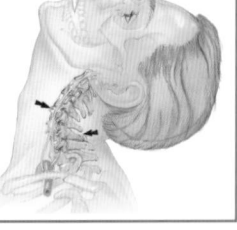

Whiplash injuries *(continued)*

Clinical tip

In all suspected spinal injuries, assume that the spine is injured until proven otherwise. Any patient with suspected whiplash or other injuries requires careful transportation from the accident scene. To do this, place him in a supine position on a spine board and immobilize his neck with tape and a hard cervical collar or sandbags.

Until an X-ray rules out a cervical fracture, move the patient as little as possible. Before the X-ray is taken, carefully remove any ear and neck jewelry. Don't undress the patient; cut clothes away, if necessary. Warn him against movements that could injure his spine.

Suicide warning signs

Watch for these warning signs of impending suicide:

- withdrawal or social isolation
- signs of depression, which may include crying, fatigue, helplessness, hopelessness, poor concentration, reduced interest in sex and other activities, sadness, constipation, and weight loss
- farewells to friends and family
- putting affairs in order
- giving away prized possessions
- expression of covert suicide messages and death wishes
- obvious suicide messages such as "I'd be better off dead."

Answering a threat

If a patient shows signs of impending suicide, assess the seriousness of the intent and the immediacy of the risk. Consider a patient with a chosen method who plans to commit suicide in the next 48 to 72 hours a high risk.

Tell the patient that you're concerned. Urge him to avoid self-destructive behavior until the staff has an opportunity to help him. Consult with the treatment team about psychiatric hospitalization.

Initiate the following safety precautions for those at high risk for suicide:

- Provide a safe environment.
- Remove dangerous objects, such as belts, razors, suspenders, electric cords, glass, knives, nail files, and clippers.
- Make the patient's specific restrictions clear to staff members, and plan for observation of the patient.
- Be alert when the patient is shaving, taking medication, or using the bathroom.
- Encourage continuity of care and consistency of primary nurses.

Normal heart rates in children

Age	Awake (beats/min)	Asleep (beats/min)	Exercise or fever (beats/min)
Neonate	100-160	80-140	< 220
1 wk-3 mo	100-220	80-200	< 220
3 mo-2 yr	80-150	70-120	< 200
2-10 yr	70-110	60-90	< 200
> 10 yr	55-100	50-90	< 200

Normal BP in children

Age	Weight (kg)	Systolic BP (mm Hg)	Diastolic BP (mm Hg)
Neonate	1	40-60	20-36
Neonate	2-3	50-70	30-45
1 mo	4	64-96	30-62
6 mo	7	60-118	50-70
1 yr	10	66-126	41-91
2-3 yr	12-14	74-124	39-89
4-5 yr	16-18	79-119	45-85
6-8 yr	20-26	80-124	45-85
10-12 yr	32-42	85-135	55-88
>14 yr	>50	90-140	60-90

Adapting injections for children

When giving an I.M. injection to a child, you'll need to adapt your approach to accommodate the child's age, the injection site, and the volume of drug you need to give. Use the table below as a guide.

Injection site	Guidelines
Deltoid	• Not recommended for children under age 3. • May be used to give 0.5 ml or less to children ages 18 mo to 3 yr if no other site is available. • Give 0.5 ml or less to children ages 3 to 15. • Give 1 ml or less to patients age 15 to adulthood.
Gluteus maximus or ventrogluteal site	• Not recommended for children under age 3. • May be used to give 1 ml or less to children ages 18 mo to 3 yr if no other site is available. • Give 1.5 ml or less to children ages 3 to 6. • Give 2 ml or less to children ages 6 to 15. • Give 2.5 ml or less to patients age 15 to adulthood.
Vastus lateralis or rectus femoris	• Give 1 ml or less to children under age 3. • Give 1.5 ml or less to children ages 3 to 6. • Give 2 ml or less to children ages 6 to 15. • Give 2.5 ml or less to patients age 15 to adulthood.

Broselow Emergency Tape

The Broselow pediatric color-coded resuscitation tape is used in the emergency assessment of children. The tape quickly indexes infant and child weight, drug dosage, and equipment and includes precalculated resuscitation drug infusion rates and CPR standards. Because indexing is based on the child's length, proper use of the tape is essential.

• Extend the Broselow tape so that the multicolor weight side is visible.

• Ensure that the tape has no bends or wrinkles.

• Place the red end of the tape even with the top of the infant's or child's head.

• Place one hand at the top of the tape, with the edge of your hand resting in the red box at the end of the tape.

• Run your free hand down the tape from the patient's head to his lower extremities (you may need someone to help you if you can't reach the lower part of the child's body).

• Stop at the patient's heel. Do not measure to the toes.

• The edge of your free hand that lands on the tape adjacent to the patient's heels indicates the patient's weight in kilograms and the patient's color zone.

• Verbalize out loud and document the color zone and the weight of the child.

• For children longer than measureable on the tape, don't use the tape; proceed as you would with an adult patient.

• Use the pediatric resuscitation supplies in the drawer of the pediatric emergency cart with the same color zone.

Recognizing child abuse and neglect

If you suspect that a child is being harmed, contact your local child protective services or the police. Contact the Childhelp USA National Child Abuse Hotline (1-800-4-A-CHILD) to find out where and how to file a report.

The following signs may indicate child abuse or neglect.

The child

- Shows sudden changes in behavior or school performance
- Hasn't received help for physical or medical problems brought to the parent's attention
- Is always watchful, as if preparing for something bad to happen
- Lacks adult supervision
- Is overly compliant, passive, or withdrawn
- Comes to school or activities early, stays late, and doesn't want to go home

The parent

- Shows little concern for the child
- Denies or blames the child for the child's problems in school or at home
- Requests that teachers or caregivers use harsh physical discipline if the child misbehaves
- Sees the child as entirely bad, worthless, or burdensome
- Demands a level of physical or academic performance the child can't achieve
- Looks primarily to the child for care, attention, and satisfaction of emotional needs

The parent and child

- Rarely look at each other
- Consider their relationship to be entirely negative
- State that they don't like each other

Assessing pregnancy information

GTPAL

Gravida = number of pregnancies, including present one
Term = total number of infants born at term, or at 37 or more weeks
Preterm = total number of infants born before 37 weeks
Abortions = total number of spontaneous or induced abortions
Living = total number of children still living

Assessing gestational age

Nägele's rule: First day of last menses minus (−) 3 months plus (+) 7 days = estimated date of delivery

Danger signs of pregnancy

• Severe vomiting
• Frequent, severe headaches
• Epigastric pain
• Fluid discharge from vagina
• Fetal movement changes or cessation after quickening
• Swelling of fingers or face
• Vision disturbances
• Signs of vaginal or urinary tract infections
• Unusual or severe abdominal pain
• Seizures or muscular irritability
• Preterm signs of labor, such as rhythmic contractions

True vs. false labor

True labor

• Regular contractions
• Back discomfort that spreads to the abdomen
• Progressive cervical dilation and effacement
• Gradually shorter intervals between contractions
• Increased intensity of contractions during ambulation
• Contractions that increase in duration and intensity

False labor

• Irregular contractions
• Discomfort that's localized in the abdomen
• No cervical change
• No change or irregular change in intervals between contractions
• Contractions may be relieved by ambulation
• Usually no change in contractions

Special

Fetal monitoring terminology

Baseline fetal heart rate (FHR): Average FHR over two contraction cycles or 10 minutes

Baseline changes: Fluctuations in FHR unrelated to uterine contractions

Periodic changes: Fluctuations in FHR related to uterine contractions

Amplitude: Difference in beats per minute between baseline readings and fluctuations in FHR

Recovery time: Difference between the end of the contraction and the return to baseline FHR

Acceleration: Transient rise in FHR lasting longer than 15 seconds and associated with a uterine contraction

Deceleration: Transient fall in FHR related to a uterine contraction

Lag time: Difference between the peak of the contraction and the lowest point of deceleration

Conditions requiring immediate cesarean section

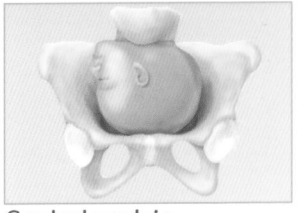

Fetal malpresentation

• May be cephalic (head first), breech (buttocks or feet first), or shoulder (shoulder, iliac crest, hand, or elbow first)

• Increases risk of complications to mother and fetus

Cephalopelvic disproportion

• Disproportion of fetal head to maternal pelvis diameter

• Labor fails to progress

• May result in malpositioning

• May result in cord prolapse if membranes rupture

Conditions requiring immediate cesarean section (continued)

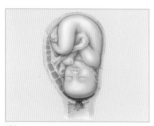

Placenta previa
- Placenta implanted in lower uterine segment
- Placenta may encroach, partially occlude, or completely occlude cervical os
- Painless, bright red, episodic vaginal bleeding after 20th week
- Soft, nontender uterus
- Fetal malpresentation

- Cord may be compressed, compromising circulation to fetus

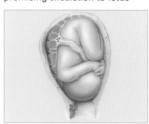

Abruptio placentae
- Premature separation of placenta from uterine wall (mild, moderate, or severe)
- Most common in multigravidas after 24 weeks
- Heavy maternal bleeding; if severe, may lead to shock and fetal death

Fetal distress
- Bradycardia
- Tachycardia
- Late or variable decelerations

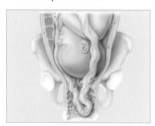

Umbilical cord prolapse
- Descent of umbilical cord into vagina before fetus

Elder abuse

Use the following guidelines to help evaluate the possibility of abuse of an older adult.

Assessment

- Burns
- Physical or thermal injury on head, face, or scalp
- Bruises and hematomas (unusual location, bruise in the shape of fingerprints, presence of other injuries in different stages of resolution)
- Mental status and neurologic changes
- Fractures, falls, or evidence of physical restraint (such as contractures)
- Ambulation status (poor ambulation or trouble sitting may suggest sexual assault)

Documentation

- Size, shape, and location of injury
- If no new lesions appear during patient's hospitalization
- If family or caregivers don't visit or show concern
- Abnormal or suspicious behavior of the older person (extremely agitated, fearful, or overly quiet and passive; fearful of caregiver)
- Patient-caregiver interaction

Vital signs

Vital sign ranges vary from neonates to older adults, as shown in the chart below.

Age	Temperature °Fahrenheit	Temperature °Celsius	Pulse rate (beats/min)	Respiratory rate (breaths/min)	Blood pressure (mm Hg)
Neonate	98.6 to 99.8	37 to 37.7	100 to 160	30 to 50	73/45
3 yr	98.5 to 99.5	36.9 to 37.5	80 to 125	20 to 30	90/55
10 yr	97.5 to 98.6	36.4 to 37	70 to 110	16 to 22	96/57
16 yr	97.6 to 98.8	36.4 to 37.1	55 to 100	15 to 20	120/80
Adult	96.8 to 99.5	36 to 37.5	60 to 100	12 to 20	120/80
Older adult	96.5 to 97.5	35.8 to 36.4	60 to 100	15 to 25	120/80

Temperature conversion

Use these formulas to convert temperatures from Fahrenheit (F) to Celsius (C) or Celsius to Fahrenheit.

$$(F - 32) \div 1.8 = \text{degrees Celsius}$$
$$(C \times 1.8) + 32 = \text{degrees Fahrenheit}$$

Resource

Height and weight conversions

Height conversion

To convert a patient's height from inches to centimeters, multiply the number of inches by 2.54. To convert a patient's height from centimeters to inches, multiply the number of centimeters by 0.394.

Imperial	Inches	Metric (cm)
4'8"	56	142
4'9"	57	144.5
4'10"	58	147
4'11"	59	150
5'	60	152.5
5'1"	61	155
5'2"	62	157.5
5'3"	63	160
5'4"	64	162.5
5'5"	65	165
5'6"	66	167.5
5'7"	67	170
5'8"	68	172.5
5'9"	69	175
5'10"	70	177.5
5'11"	71	180
6'	72	183
6'1"	73	185.5
6'2"	74	188
6'3"	75	190.5

Weight conversion

To convert a patient's weight from pounds to kilograms, divide the number of pounds by 2.2 kg; to convert a patient's weight from kilograms to pounds, multiply the number of kilograms by 2.2 lb.

Pounds	Kilograms
10	4.5
20	9
30	13.6
40	18.1
50	22.7
60	27.2
70	31.8
80	36.3
90	40.9
100	45.4
110	49.9
120	54.4
130	59
140	63.5
150	68
160	72.6
170	77.1
180	81.6
190	86.2
200	90.8
210	95.5
220	100
230	104.5
240	109.1
250	113.6
260	118.2

Adult immunization schedule

The immunization schedule below is recommended for adults older than age 18.

Vaccine	Timing and considerations
Hepatitis A for those at risk	Two doses 6 to 12 months apart to provide long-term protection; first dose 4 weeks before departure to endemic countries
Hepatitis B if never had initial series	Three doses: second dose at least 1 month after first; third dose 5 months after first dose
Measles, mumps, and rubella	Two doses 1 month apart if born after 1957 and immunity can't be proved; contraindicated in pregnancy, cancer, immunosuppression, and HIV infection
Tetanus-diphtheria if never had initial series	Three doses: second dose 1 month after first; third dose 6 to 12 months after second; booster for all patients every 10 years
Varicella-zoster	Two doses for susceptible adults who haven't had chickenpox; second dose 1 month after first; contraindicated in pregnancy, cancer, immunosuppression, and HIV infection
Influenza	Annually before flu season (September to December in the United States), especially for those age 65 and older; those with heart or lung disease, diabetes, or other chronic conditions; and those who work or live with high-risk individuals
Pneumococcal	One dose at age 65; also recommended for persons with chronic disease (see indications for influenza) and those with kidney disorders or sickle cell anemia; possibly a repeat dose 5 years later for those at highest risk; may be given any time of the year

Adapted from the U.S. Department of Health and Human Services, U.S. Preventative Services Task Force (2003).

Childhood immunization schedule

This schedule shows the recommended ages for routine administration of childhood vaccines, as approved by the CDC in 2005. Note that new recommendations for hepatitis A are pending.

Vaccine / Age	Birth	1 mo	2 mo	4 mo	6 mo	12 mo	15 mo	18 mo	24 mo	4-6 yr	11-12 yr	13-18 yr
Hepatitis B (HepB)	HepB #1	HepB #2			HepB #3						HepB series	
Diphtheria, tetanus, pertussis (DTaP)			DTaP	DTaP	DTaP			DTaP		DTaP	Td	Td
Haemophilus influenzae type b (Hib)			Hib	Hib	Hib	Hib						
Inactivated poliovirus (IPV)			IPV	IPV	IPV					IPV		
Measles, mumps, rubella (MMR)						MMR #1				MMR #2	MMR #2	
Varicella						Varicella				Varicella		
Pneumococcal (PCV)			PCV	PCV	PCV	PCV			PCV	PPV		
Influenza					Influenza (yearly for selected populations)	Influenza (yearly)				Influenza (yearly)		
Hepatitis A										Hepatitis A series		

Vaccines below dotted line are for selected populations

Key:
- Range of recommended ages
- Preadolescent assessment
- Only if mother is HBsAg-negative
- Catch-up vaccine

Catch-up immunization schedule

The next two charts show schedules and minimum intervals between doses for children who have delayed immunizations.

For children ages 4 months to 6 years

Vaccine	Minimum age for dose 1	Minimum interval between doses			
		Dose 1 to dose 2	Dose 2 to dose 3	Dose 3 to dose 4	Dose 4 to dose 5
Diphtheria, tetanus, pertussis	6 wk	4 wk	4 wk	6 mo	6 mo
Inactivated poliovirus	6 wk	4 wk	4 wk	4 wk	
Hepatitis B	Birth	4 wk	8 wk (and 16 wk after first dose)		
Measles, mumps, rubella (MMR)	12 mo	4 wk			
Varicella	12 mo				
Haemophilus influenzae type b	6 wk	• 4 wk (if first dose at age <12 mo) • 8 wk (as final dose if first dose at age 12-14 mo)	• 4 wk (if current age is <12 mo) • 8 wk (as final dose if current age is ≥12 mo and second dose at age <15 mo)	8 wk (as final dose; only necessary for children age 12 mo-5 yr who received 3 doses before age 12 mo)	

(continued)

For children ages 4 months to 6 years (continued)

Vaccine	Minimum age for dose 1	Minimum interval between doses			
		Dose 1 to dose 2	Dose 2 to dose 3	Dose 3 to dose 4	Dose 4 to dose 5
Pneumococcal	6 wk	• 4 wk (if first dose at age < 12 mo and current age is < 24 mo) • 8 wk (as final dose if first dose at age ≥ 12 mo or current age is 24 to 59 mo)	• 4 wk (if current age < 12 mo) • 8 wk (as final dose if current age ≥ 12 mo)	8 wk (as final dose; only necessary for children age 12 mo to 5 yr who received 3 doses before age 12 mo)	

For children ages 7 to 18 years

Vaccine	Minimum interval between doses		
	Dose 1 to dose 2	Dose 2 to dose 3	Dose 3 to booster dose
Tetanus, diphtheria	4 wk	6 mo	• 6 mo (if first dose at age < 12 mo and current age is < 11 yr) • 5 yr (if first dose at age ≥ 12 mo, third dose at age < 7 yr, and current age is ≥ 11 yr) • 10 yr (if third dose at age ≥ 7 yr)
Inactivated poliovirus	4 wk	4 wk	
Hepatitis B	4 wk	8 wk (and 16 wk after first dose)	
MMR	4 wk		
Varicella	4 wk		

Treatment for biological weapons exposure

Listed below are potentially threatening biological (bacterial and viral) agents as well as treatments and vaccines currently available.

Implement standard precautions for all cases of suspected exposure. For cases of smallpox, institute airborne precautions for the duration of the illness and until all scabs fall off. For pneumonic plague cases, institute droplet precautions for 72 hours after initiation of effective therapy.

Biological agent (condition)	Treatment
Bacillus anthracis (anthrax)	• Ciprofloxacin, doxycycline, or penicillin • Vaccine: Limited supply available; not recommended in absence of exposure to anthrax
Clostridium botulinum (botulism)	• Supportive: ET intubation and mechanical ventilation • Passive immunization with equine antitoxin to lessen nerve damage • Vaccine: Postexposure prophylaxis with equine botulinum antitoxin; botulinum toxoid available from CDC; recombinant vaccine under development
Francisella tularensis (tularemia)	• Gentamicin or streptomycin; alternatively, doxycycline, chloramphenicol, or ciprofloxacin • Vaccine: Live, attenuated vaccine currently under investigation and review by the Food and Drug Administration (FDA)
Variola major (smallpox)	• No FDA-approved antiviral available; cidofovir may be therapeutic if administered 1 to 2 days after exposure • Vaccine: Prophylaxis within 3 to 4 days of exposure
Yersinia pestis (pneumonic plague)	• Streptomycin or gentamicin; alternatively, doxycycline, ciprofloxacin, or chloramphenicol • Vaccine: No longer available

Assessing brain death

Only a doctor or coroner may legally pronounce a person dead. Criteria for determining brain death vary, but the following are commonly used:

• Patient is unresponsive to all stimuli.
• Pupillary responses are absent.
• All brain functions cease.
• No eye movements are noted when cold water is instilled into ears (caloric test). Normally, eyes move toward irrigated ear.
• No corneal reflex is present.
• No gag reflex is present.
• Quick rotation of patient's head from left to right (doll's eyes test) causes eyes to remain fixed, suggesting brain death. Normally, eyes move in the opposite direction of head movement.
• Apnea test reveals no spontaneous breathing.
• EEG shows no brain activity or response.
• If the patient is declared brain dead, organ and tissue donation may be discussed with the family, unless precluding conditions exist (such as cancer, HIV, AIDS, or advanced age). Family consent must be obtained for tissue and organ harvesting.

Reportable situations in the ED

Reportable situation	Agency
Homicide	• Coroner • Law enforcement
Suicide	• Coroner • Law enforcement
Altercations and assaults	• Law enforcement
Motor vehicle crashes	• Law enforcement
Deaths	• Coroner • Local organ procurement agency (in most states)
Child abuse	• Child protective services
Elder abuse	• Adult protective services
Communicable diseases	• Varies by state
Animal bites	• Animal control

Telephone triage

Telephone triage involves clinicians taking telephone calls and processing requests for medical advice or services.

Who may take the call?

Experienced professional RNs with specialized education in triage, telephone assessment, communication, and documentation

Rules of telephone triage

- Introduce yourself and establish rapport with the caller.
- Obtain baseline information.
- Obtain demographic data.
- Obtain important times:
  - when caller phoned service or hospital
  - when triage nurse began speaking to caller
  - time call finished
  - notification of 911, doctor, and ED.
- Get adequate information before giving advice to the patient.
- Make a triage decision using established protocols or guidelines of your institution. (If a doctor backup is available, you may choose to review the call with the doctor first.)
- Offer only the predetermined (by the institution's established protocols) advice.
- Conclude the call and follow up as needed.
- Document all information precisely, including recommendations or protocols used and follow-up measures.
- When faced with calls needing advanced or basic life support, instruct the caller to call 911 or to go to the nearest ED.

Protocols

- Facility must have step-by-step protocols on how to manage calls, based on symptoms or diagnosis.
- Protocols may be original or purchased outside.
- Doctors in the practice must approve protocols.
- You must have the doctor's approval for prescriptive protocols.
- All advice or instruction to patient must follow the doctor's directions or orders.
- Standing orders for specific, recurring issues are acceptable only if approved by the patient's doctor.
- If medical assessment is required, a registered nurse or doctor must take the call.

EMTALA

In 1988, Congress passed the Emergency Medical Treatment and Active Labor Act (EMTALA). This act states that any patient who comes to the ED requesting examination or treatment for a medical condition must be provided with an appropriate medical screening examination to determine if he is suffering from an emergency medical condition. If he is, then the hospital is obligated to either provide him with treatment until he's stable or transfer him to another hospital in conformance with the statute's directives.

If the patient doesn't have an emergency medical condition, EMTALA imposes no further obligation on the hospital. The statute also applies to hospital inpatients, but only to those with emergency conditions.

Other provisions of EMTALA include:
• Hospitals are required to maintain a list of doctors who are on call to provide treatment to stabilize a patient with an emergency medical condition.
• If an individual with an emergency medical condition is admitted from the ED in order to stabilize the condition, the hospital has satisfied its responsibilities.
• The hospital can't admit a patient intending not to treat him and then inappropriately transfer or discharge him.
• The hospital can't delay screening or stabilization to inquire about a patient's method of payment.

Basic English-Spanish translations

English	Spanish
My name is _____	Mi nombre es _____
I am your nurse.	Soy su enfermero(a)
Come in, please.	Entre, por favor.
What is your name?	¿Cómo se llama?
How are you feeling?	¿Cómo se siente?
How old are you?	¿Cuántos años tiene?
Do you live alone?	¿Vive solo(a)?
Do you take any medications?	¿Toma medicamentos?
Are you allergic to any medications?	¿Es usted alérgico(a) a algún medicamento?
Who is your doctor?	¿Quién es su médico?
Are you comfortable?	¿Está cómodo(a)?
Do you follow a special diet?	¿Tiene Ud. una dieta especial?

pain   dolor

mild	bothersome	throbbing	intense
leve	molesto	pulsante	intenso

I would like to give you:
- an injection.
- an I.V. medication.
- a liquid medication.
- a medicated cream or powder.
- a medication through your epidural catheter.
- a medication through your rectum.
- a medication through your _____ tube.
- a medication under your tongue.
- some pill(s).
- a suppository.

Quisiera darle a Ud. un(a):
- inyección.
- medicamento por vía intravenosa.
- medicamento en forma líquida.
- medicamento en pomada o polvo.
- medicamento por el catéter epidural.
- medicamento por el recto.
- medicamento por su _____ tubo.
- medicamento debajo de la lengua.
- píldoras.
- supositorio.

Cultural considerations in patient care

As a health care professional, you'll interact with a diverse, multicultural patient population. Each culture has its own set of beliefs about health and illness, dietary practices, and other matters that you need to be familiar with when providing care.

Health and illness philosophy	Dietary practices	Other considerations
African Americans		
• May believe illness is related to supernatural causes, such as punishment from God or an evil spell • Believe health is a feeling of well-being • May seek advice and remedies from faith or folk healers	• May have food restrictions based on religious beliefs, such as not eating pork if Muslim • May view cooked greens as good for health	• Tend to be affectionate, as shown by touching and hugging friends and loved ones • If Muslim, must have head covered at all times • Respect elders, especially for their wisdom • Primary religions: Baptist, other Protestant denominations, Muslim
Arab Americans		
• Believe health is a gift from God and that one should care for oneself by eating right and minimizing stressors • May believe illness is caused by the evil eye, bad luck, stress, or an imbalance between hot and cold or moist and dry • May use amulets to ward off evil eye during illness	• Don't mix milk and fish, sweet and sour, or hot and cold • Don't use ice in drinks; believe hot soup can help recovery • If Muslim, prohibited from drinking alcohol and eating pork or ham	• Respect elders and professionals • Traditional women may avoid eye contact with male strangers • Use same-sex family members as interpreters • Primary religions: Muslim, Christian (Greek Orthodox, Protestant)

Health and illness philosophy	Dietary practices	Other considerations
Arab Americans (continued)		
• May assume passive role as patient • Believe in complete rest and ridding self of all responsibilities during illness • May have low pain threshold and express pain vocally		
Chinese Americans		
• Believe health is a balance of the principles of *yin* and *yang* and that illness stems from an imbalance of these elements; believe good health requires harmony between body, mind, and spirit • May use herbalists or acupuncturists before seeking medical help; ginseng root is a common home remedy • May use good luck objects, such as jade or rope tied around waist • Family expected to take care of patient, who assumes a passive role • Tend not to readily express pain; stoic by nature	• Rice, noodles, and vegetables are staples; tend to use chopsticks • Choose foods to help balance the *yin* (cold) and *yang* (hot) • Drink hot liquids, especially when sick	• Health care providers should keep a comfortable distance when approaching patient. • Elders should not be addressed by first name (a sign of disrespect). • Lack of eye contact may be a sign of respect. • Tend to be very modest; best to use same-sex clinicians • Primary religions: Buddhist, Catholic, Protestant

(continued)

Health and illness philosophy	Dietary practices	Other considerations
Japanese Americans		
• Believe that health is a balance of oneself, society, and the universe • May believe illness is related to karma, resulting from behavior in present or past life • May believe certain food combinations cause illness • May use prayer beads if Buddhist • May use tea to treat GI ailments and constipation • May not complain of symptoms until severe	• Eat rice with most meals; may use chopsticks • Diet high in salt; low in sugar, fat, protein, and cholesterol	• Usually quiet and polite; may ask few questions about care, deferring to health care providers • Elderly may nod but not necessarily understand • Very modest; tend to avoid touching; best to use same-sex clinicians • Primary religions: Buddhist, Shinto, Christian
Mexican Americans		
• Believe that health is influenced by environment, fate, and God's will • May believe in Galen's theory that the body's four humors — blood, phlegm, yellow bile, and black bile — must be kept in balance • May use herbal teas and soup to aid in recuperation • May self-medicate because prescription drug sales are not controlled in Mexico	• Beans and tortillas are staples • Eat lots of fresh fruits and vegetables	• Modest, especially women • Use same-sex family members as interpreters • Primary religion: Roman Catholic

Cultural considerations in patient care
(continued)

Health and illness philosophy	Dietary practices	Other considerations
Mexican Americans (continued)		
• May express pain by non-verbal cues • Family may want to keep seriousness of illness from patient		
Native Americans		
• Use herbs and roots; each tribe has its own unique medicinal practices • Typically use modern medicine where available • Use ancient symbol of Medicine Wheel • May consider number 4 sacred (associated with four primary laws of creation: life, unity, equality, and eternity) • Use tobacco for important religious, ceremonial, and medicinal purposes; may sprinkle it around patient's bed to protect and heal him	• Have balanced diet of seafood, fruits, greens, corn, rice, and garden vegetables; low in salt • Specific dietary practices based on location: Urban dwellers often eat meat, while rural residents may consume only lamb and goat	• Clan and tribe considered extended family • Elders respected • May be uncomfortable sharing their belief systems • Use "talking circle" to share information and support and to solve problems

Common abbreviations

ABG	arterial blood gas
ACE	angiotensin-converting enzyme
ACLS	advanced cardiac life support
AED	automated external defibrillator
AIDS	acquired immunodeficiency syndrome
b.i.d.	twice a day
BMI	body mass index
BP	blood pressure
CAD	coronary artery disease
CBC	complete blood count
CDC	Centers for Disease Control and Prevention
CMV	cytomegalovirus
CO	cardiac output
CO_2	carbon dioxide
COPD	chronic obstructive pulmonary disease
CPR	cardiopulmonary resuscitation
CrCl	creatinine clearance
CSF	cerebrospinal fluid
CV	cardiovascular
CVA	cerebrovascular accident
DIC	disseminated intravascular coagulation
DTR	deep tendon reflex
DVT	deep vein thrombosis
ED	emergency department
ET	endotracheal
GI	gastrointestinal
gtt	drop
GU	genitourinary
GYN	gynecologic
Hct	hematocrit
HF	heart failure
Hgb	hemoglobin
HIV	human immunodeficiency virus
hr	hour
HSV	herpes simplex virus
ICP	intracranial pressure
I.M.	intramuscular
INR	International Normalized Ratio
IOP	intraocular pressure

IPPB	intermittent positive-pressure breathing
I.V.	intravenous
LOC	level of consciousness
LR	lactated Ringer's (solution)
MAO	monoamine oxidase
MI	myocardial infarction
min	minute
ml	milliliter
NaCl	sodium chloride
NG	nasogastric
NIH	National Institutes of Health
NSAID	nonsteroidal anti-inflammatory drug
O_2	oxygen
OCD	obsessive-compulsive disorder
OTC	over-the-counter
$Paco_2$	partial pressure of carbon dioxide in arterial blood
Pao_2	partial pressure of oxygen in arterial blood
PEA	pulseless electrical activity
PID	pelvic inflammatory disease
PIH	pregnancy-induced hypertension
P.O.	by mouth
P.R.	by rectum
p.r.n.	as needed
q	every
q.i.d.	four times a day
sec	second
S.L.	sublingual
SSRI	selective serotonin reuptake inhibitor
subQ	subcutaneous
TB	tuberculosis
TCA	tricyclic antidepressant
t.i.d.	three times a day
TPN	total parenteral nutrition
trach	tracheostomy
UTI	urinary tract infection
VF	ventricular fibrillation
VT	ventricular tachycardia
wt	weight

Index

Selected references

Bickley, L.S., and Szilagyi, P.G. *Bates' Guide to Physical Examination and History Taking*, 8th ed. Philadelphia: Lippincott Williams & Wilkins, 2003.

Briggs, J.K., and Grossman, V.G. *Emergency Nursing: 5-Tier Triage Protocols.* Philadelphia: Lippincott Williams & Wilkins, 2006.

ECG Interpretation: An Incredibly Easy Pocket Guide. Philadelphia: Lippincott Williams & Wilkins, 2006.

Fischbach, F. *A Manual of Laboratory and Diagnostic Tests*, 7th ed. Philadelphia: Lippincott Williams & Wilkins, 2004.

Fultz, J., and Sturt, P. *Mosby's Emergency Nursing Reference*, 3rd ed. Philadelphia: Mosby, 2005.

Grossman, V.G.A. *Quick Reference to Triage*, 2nd ed. Philadelphia: Lippincott Williams & Wilkins, 2003.

Hazinski, M.F., et al., eds. *Handbook of Emergency Cardiovascular Care for Healthcare Providers.* Dallas: American Heart Association, 2004.

Mastering ACLS, 2nd ed. Philadelphia: Lippincott Williams & Wilkins, 2006.

Newberry, L. et al., eds. *Sheehy's Emergency Nursing*, 6th ed. Philadelphia: W.B. Saunders, 2005.

Nursing2006 Drug Handbook, 26th ed. Philadelphia: Lippincott Williams & Wilkins, 2006.

Proehl, J.A. *Emergency Nursing Procedures*, 3rd ed. Philadelphia: W.B. Saunders, 2004.

ER Facts Made Incredibly Quick!

- ◆ Triage assessments and acuity systems
- ◆ Laboratory values
- ◆ CPR and ACLS guidelines
- ◆ ECG monitoring
- ◆ Medication administration guidelines and tools
- ◆ Nursing considerations for common ER conditions, including burns, fractures, and trauma
- ◆ Guidelines for special patient populations
- ◆ English-Spanish translations
- ◆ Color-coded tabs that help you find information fast
- ◆ Write-on, waterproof pages that come clean with an alcohol wipe

Other Incredibly Quick titles

- ◆ *Drug Facts Made Incredibly Quick*
- ◆ *ECG Facts Made Incredibly Quick*
- ◆ *ICU/CCU Facts Made Incredibly Quick*
- ◆ *LPN Facts Made Incredibly Quick*
- ◆ *Maternal-Neonatal Facts Made Incredibly Quick*
- ◆ *Nursing Facts Made Incredibly Quick*
- ◆ *Pediatric Facts Made Incredibly Quick*
- ◆ *Wound Care Facts Made Incredibly Quick*

ISBN 1-58255-591-5

90000>

9 781582 555911

Nursing Category:
Emergency Care